INDIVIDUAL LIBERTY AND MEDICAL CONTROL

Individual Liberty and Medical Control

HETA HÄYRY

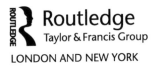

Routledge
Taylor & Francis Group

LONDON AND NEW YORK

First published 1998 by Ashgate Publishing

Reissued 2018 by Routledge
2 Park Square, Milton Park, Abingdon, Oxon, OX14 4RN
711 Third Avenue, New York, NY 10017, USA

Routledge is an imprint of the Taylor & Francis Group, an informa business

Publisher's Note
The publisher has gone to great lengths to ensure the quality of this reprint but points out that some imperfections in the original copies may be apparent.

Disclaimer
The publisher has made every effort to trace copyright holders and welcomes correspondence from those they have been unable to contact.

A Library of Congress record exists under LC control number: 98073764

ISBN 13: 978-1-138-32040-6 (hbk)
ISBN 13: 978-0-429-45329-8 (ebk)

Contents

Acknowledgements

The themes of this book, the philosophical and practical questions regarding individual liberty and medical control, have occupied my mind for the last decade or so. I have occasionally had the opportunity to deal with some of the issues over the years, but I have not previously had the chance to bring all my thoughts together in book form. It is therefore with gratitude that I acknowledge the financial support, in the form of a Senior Research Fellowship, of the Academy of Finland which has made it possible for me to complete this volume.

I have discussed the topics covered in this book with many friends and colleagues to whom I would like to extend my thanks. Of the persons who are in one way or another the most directly responsible for the existence, if not the content, of these chapters I must single out Timo Airaksinen, John Harris, Søren Holm and Matti Häyry. More specific expressions of gratitude have been included, where appropriate, in the notes of the individual chapters.

Heta Häyry
Helsinki, February 1997

Introduction: The Nature, Value and Limits of Individual Liberty

Bioethics as an academic discipline consists of a variety of scholarly attempts to deal with the moral, social and political problems emerging from the practice of healing and caring, biomedical research and the provision of health care services. The primary aim of many professional bioethicists is, of late, to *solve*, as efficiently as possible, the problems encountered by health care providers and scientists in clinical, laboratory and administrative settings. Seen from the viewpoint of applied philosophy, however, this is a dangerous tendency if the *grounds* for the suggested solutions are not properly examined. Even choices which are harmless and seem to involve no immoralities can be indirectly hazardous if those making the choices appeal to dubious ethical principles or inaccurate data.[1] This is why this book is dedicated to the examination of the *reasons* that people can and should have for their health-care related decisions as well as to the formulation of good solutions to difficult problems.

The theoretical questions which are characteristic to bioethics always have a practical slant, but they are often also connected with deep metaphysical issues which lie at the core of various ethical doctrines. The most important questions concern the value of life, the role of expertise in medical decision-making and conflicts between various moral claims.

The definition, value and meaning of human life have been central in debates regarding abortion, euthanasia and genetic engineering. The relevant questions include the following. When does a new human life come into being? What gives a human life its worth? Are some lives more – or less – worth living than others? When does a human life end? How should we treat entities which could become, or have once been, living human beings?

Some philosophers have thought that these questions can be best answered by referring to the doctrine of the sanctity of life, or by reference to the biological, social or metaphysical potential shared by certain living beings.[2] Those who have assumed this manner of thinking have usually contended that it would be morally wrong to terminate a pregnancy or to give a lethal injection to a terminal patient who wants to die quickly and without excessive pain. This would, they can argue, violate the sanctity of human life. Alternatively, they can say that practices like these would deny or prevent the

1

realization, or actualization, of some of the potential possessed by the human beings whose lives are interfered with.

Other philosophers, in contrast, have maintained that the proper criterion for defining the beginning and the end of ethically meaningful human life can be found by focusing on consciousness, and that under most circumstances the best way to measure the value of individual human lives is to consult the individuals themselves.[3]

The first part of this view is based on the observation that most adult human beings are aware of their own continued existence as subjects of beliefs, expectations, hopes, fears and other mental states. If the hopes and expectations of these individuals to continue their existence are frustrated by taking their lives, they are obviously wronged by the deed. But the situation can be different when it comes to beings who have never been, or will never again become, aware of themselves as subjects of mental states. According to the consciousness view, individuals like these cannot be genuinely wronged by terminating their lives, and this is why abortion – along with decisions not to keep irreversibly comatose patients alive – should be morally condoned.

The second part of the view states that individuals are usually the best judges of their own lives and their own life quality. If they see their lives as good, then it is not the legitimate business of others to intervene without explicit permission. Similarly, if individuals deem their lives to be worthless, and wish to hasten their death, other people should not automatically try to keep them alive, or condemn those who are willing to help them to die quickly and easily. An important task within a view like this is, of course, to define clearly the circumstances under which individuals should be allowed to make drastic decisions concerning their own lives. According to a standard interpretation, people should not be granted the right to full self-determination if they are very young, or if they suffer from severe mental defects or senility. Furthermore, individuals should not be given a decisive say in matters which have to do with their wellbeing, if they lack sufficient psychological control over their choices due to temporary emotional disturbances, lack of knowledge, or the undue influence of other people.

All these questions, and particularly the generic question concerning the proper limits of individual liberty in health care, will be discussed in some detail in the seven chapters which constitute the corpus of this book. I shall begin in chapter 1 by examining certain hypothetical situations where a choice must be made between the lives of two separate individuals. In chapter 2 the legitimacy of hastening the death of autonomous persons at their own request will be considered, and in chapter 3 the inquiry is extended more generally to the role of people's own wishes in decisions regarding health care provision. Chapter 4 sheds light on the attitudes of medical professionals by presenting and refuting a mechanistic model of health education, and by outlining an autonomy-respecting alternative which ideally aims at rendering people aware of the conditions of their own physical health.

In chapter 5 the focus is shifted to questions in preventive medicine. Is it acceptable that the public health authorities restrict the liberty of individuals in order to promote the welfare of the population at large? The issues of medical prevention from quarantines to prescription drug laws are studied to answer this question. The theme of prevention is further explored in chapter 6, where legislation regarding persons who are HIV infected are discussed. The major view that I defend is that discrimination and legal restrictions cannot be justifiably based on the irrational and moralistic fears that people may have towards each other.

Since it is, obviously, difficult to find ethical principles that everybody can both condone and understand in the same way, the idea of democratic decision-making in medicine and health care may seem attractive. This possibility is taken up in chapter 7, where democracy in medical matters is examined in the light of the most important prevailing theories of social and political philosophy. There are two dividing lines which distinguish these theories from each other. First, some theorists maintain that freedom can be equalled with freedom from constraint, while others argue that to be genuinely free individuals must accept certain specified restrictions. Second, many philosophers have thought that people's vital needs ought to be satisfied regardless of their merits, while others have disagreed. In the concluding chapter of this book I defend a model which I call liberal egalitarian, and which combines an antipaternalistic concept of liberty with the demand that people ought to be helped when they are in need. Certain elements of this view will already be delineated and defended in this introductory chapter.

The topics that I have chosen for my book are designed to bring to the fore some of the most important questions related to the theme of individual liberty and medical control in bioethics. The elementary life-and-death situations introduced in the first chapter provide me with a framework for considering what human life is and what gives it its value. These questions are further studied in the chapters dealing with voluntary euthanasia, forms of medical authoritarianism, and health education. In these reflections, as well as in the sections on preventive medicine and AIDS, the conflicts between people's attitudes, interests and needs are also central to my analysis. In the final chapter the suggested solutions to the problems of medical responsibility and individual liberty are classified according to the political and ideological assumptions which can be found at the foundations of mutually contradictory views on bioethics.

Since this is a book mainly on the applications of philosophy to the questions related to liberty and medical control, it is, I believe, necessary that I briefly describe the theoretical considerations which underlie my more practical views. The most significant of these concern the nature and value of individual freedom and self-determination, but I shall also extend my preliminary normative remarks and methodological comments to the principles of wellbeing, happiness and justice.

Liberal thinkers have usually defined freedom either as the lack of constraints or as the ability of individuals to decide for themselves what happens in their lives.[4] Within the most classical forms of liberalism, to say that people are free means primarily that they are not legally or otherwise coercively prevented from acting according to their desires and plans. This definition is, however, problematical on two accounts. On the one hand, individuals are not always free, at least not according to everyday thinking, even if they are not hindered from doing what they desire, or want, to do. Persons serving a prison sentence can, under some circumstances, want to be imprisoned, but this does not liberate them in the very ordinary sense that they could walk out of the prison if they had a sudden urge to do so. On the other hand, individuals are not completely free even if they are free from coercion and deliberate constraint. Nobody actively prevents us from travelling to the sun, but we are nevertheless unable – and consequently unfree – to make the trip.

As the fulfilment of desires seems to be an inadequate basis for definitions of freedom, some theorists have referred, instead, to the non-restriction of options, or action alternatives.[5] Individuals are free to act in a specified way if they can choose to act in that way without any constraint. Restrictions of freedom can, within this view, be generated either naturally or by human actions. Prisoners cannot leave their penitentiaries and human beings cannot travel to the centre of our solar system because they cannot overcome the concrete obstacles that stand in the way of their freedom.

In addition, however, human actions can also create restrictions of an entirely different kind. Coercion which is founded on the use of credible threats does not actually prevent people from acting in the way they had planned to act, but it does nonetheless decrease their range of options. Pedestrians who are seized on the street and told that they are to surrender either their money or their lives can walk ahead without giving their money to the robber, but by doing so they risk being physically harmed. When the situation after the threat is compared to the situation preceding it, the alternative in which the pedestrians could keep both their money and their lives has ceased to exist, and this is why they are, in this particular respect, unfree.

Restrictions of freedom can influence people by being present, in which case they are technically referred to as 'positive constraints'. Examples of these are physical obstacles and violent threats. But there are also elements of unfreedom which influence individuals by their absence, and which can be called 'negative constraints'. These include, for instance, lack of money and other resources. A family without adequate financial means cannot buy an expensive house even if nobody can be blamed for deliberately preventing or hindering the purchase.[6]

Both positive and negative constraints can be further divided into the 'external' and the 'internal'.[7] Prison walls, threats and lack of money are all external obstacles which exist outside the mind-body continuums of human beings. Pains and obsessions are positive internal constraints which work by being physiologically or mentally present, while moral weakness and lack of talent are negative internal constraints which are based on the absence of certain desirable properties or character traits in human beings.

Opponents of liberalism have often argued that there are internal constraints which are in fact essential if we try to pursue our true, or 'positive freedom'.[8] According to these antiliberal thinkers, a person whose high moral standards prevent her from inflicting harm on innocent human beings is not unfree, but rather free in the most genuine and significant sense. The fact that she has become aware of the basic requirements of social life, and consequently respects them in her actions, makes her truly free. On the other hand, individuals who have not been able to learn and to internalize these rules should, so the argument goes, be regarded as unfree.

The concept of positive freedom, together with its inherent demands concerning the behaviour of individuals, is obviously illiberal. The proponents of the model believe, among other things, that individuals can be forced to be free – an idea which cannot possibly be accepted in the liberal camp. But this is not to say that moral ideals and ethical principles should always be treated as constraints on the liberty of individuals. At least those moral views which are consciously chosen by the individuals themselves can be seen to define rather than restrict their freedom. Since most people are autonomous beings, they should be allowed to determine the limits of their inner freedom on the basis of their own experiences and ideas. The person who abstains from harming others on ethical grounds is unfree to hurt others, but she can still be free to act according to her own self-determined principles.

Both the non-restriction of options and the capacity to make autonomous decisions have been seen as valuable in the liberal tradition. Some theorists have thought that the value of freedom is intrinsic and intuitively detectable to anybody. They think that it is symbolically important to individuals to know that there are more books in the nearby library than they are ever going to read, and more dishes in the menu of their neighbouring restaurant than they are ever going to order.[9] These theorists can also believe that the freedom of choice exemplified by the books and the dishes is somehow self-evidently valuable, and should in no way be restricted.

There are, however, difficulties with this argument for freedom and its intrinsic value. A wide range of choices can, of course, be symbolically exhilarating and personally satisfying, but so can military marches and psychedelic drugs. It would not be easy to build a workable system of liberties on such elusive axiological grounds.

Other champions of liberty have argued that the value of freedom is instrumental rather than intrinsic. A society, they say, which does not unduly interfere with the choices of its members encourages their creativity, genius and industriousness.[10] These qualities, theorists of this persuasion can continue, are valuable because creative and industrious individuals lay the foundation for material wellbeing and cultural flourishing in a society, and bring happiness to the nation as a whole.

The flaw of this defence is that it cannot be supported by empirical proof. Nations have been known to flourish both materially and culturally when their citizens have been strictly controlled by religious principles, and even political dictatorships have often provided the majority of their subjects good and secure living conditions.

A better way to defend the value of freedom can, I think, be found by distinguishing between two separate axiological levels as regards liberty and its affiliates. First, the value of freedom of action and freedom of choice is instrumental, and it is based on the fact that the non-restriction of a person's options is, to some degree at least, a necessary condition for autonomous decision-making. Second, autonomy and self-determination are valuable in themselves, since they belong to the primary elements of a good and happy human life. Material wellbeing is, no doubt, possible without liberty and autonomy, but whether or not such welfare is worth pursuing is another matter. The happiness that most ethical theories see as the highest goal of human life conceptually presupposes that individuals are free to decide what the direction of their life and their actions is.

If this analysis can be accepted, then the intrinsic value of autonomy guarantees that the freedom of choices and actions is instrumentally valuable to individuals who aim at making self-determined decisions. It follows from this that moral agents should try not to violate the liberty and autonomy of other agents unless they have good grounds for doing so. But as liberty and autonomy are not the only values in the universe, it seems reasonable to think that respect for them can sometimes be overridden by appeals to other worthy goals. This is why one important task for any liberal theory is to define the relationship of liberty and autonomy with the other values that people may hold dear.

John Stuart Mill formulated in the most famous passage of his essay *On Liberty* (1859) the limits of liberty as follows:

> The object of this Essay is to assert one very simple principle, as entitled to govern absolutely the dealings of the society with the individual in the way of compulsion and control, whether the means used be physical force in the form of legal penalties, or the moral coercion of public opinion. That principle is, that the sole end for which mankind are warranted, individually or collectively, in interfering with the liberty of action of any of their number, is self-protection. That the only purpose for which power can be rightfully exercised over any member of a civilized community, against his will, is to prevent harm to others. His own good, either physical or moral, is not a sufficient warrant. He cannot rightfully be compelled to do or forbear because it will be better for him to do so, because it will make him happier, because, in the opinion of others, to do so would be wise, or even right. These are good reasons for remonstrating with him, or reasoning with him, or persuading him, or entreating him, but not for compelling him, or visiting him with any evil in case he do otherwise. To justify that, the conduct from which it is desired to deter him, must be calculated to produce evil to some one else. The only part of the conduct of any one, for which he is amenable to society, is that which concerns others. In the part which merely concerns himself, his independence is, of right, absolute. Over himself, over his own body and mind, the individual is sovereign.[11]

This passage contains, in fact, an array of ethical principles which define the 'liberal utilitarianism', or 'utilitarian liberalism', professed by Mill and his followers.[12]

Mill asserted that the only good reason for permanent restrictions of liberty is the harm people can inflict on innocent, non-consenting others. Although the violations of liberty and autonomy are – even in these cases – harmful and prima facie wrong, they can be justified by appeals to the greater harm which would result from the evildoer's exercise of freedom. The harm in question can be physical or psychological, it can be inflicted directly or indirectly, and it can fall upon the victims either in one blow or gradually. Mill thought, as do his fellow utilitarians, that it is of little or no consequence whether the harm is inflicted by acting or by failing to act, as long as in both cases the quality and quantity of harm remains the same. It is, however, another matter how efficiently people can be coerced into action which is expected to benefit only or mainly others. This is why legislation is seldom the right instrument when public authorities want to enforce the positive obligations of the citizens towards each other.

When the harmful consequences of acts and omissions are assessed, everybody's desires and interests should, according to the Millian view, be considered equally.[13] Some moralists have thought that this principle of equality, or impartiality, implies that legislators and other political decision-makers ought to sacrifice the interests of minorities in order to serve the good of the majority. If everybody's vaguest hopes and desires must be taken into account with the same seriousness as somebody's survival and health, even the most unimportant desires of a very large number of individuals seem to justify the suffering and death of a few.

Whatever the official utilitarian line regarding the sacrifice of the minorities is, however, I myself prefer an interpretation which does not allow the straightforward comparison of different kinds of utilities. Surely the equal consideration of everybody's interests does not mean that the transitory pleasures of the majority should legitimize grave harm inflicted on a minority. The point of the principle is, more likely, that the less important desires of individuals must not be taken into account in the assessment of the outcomes of actions unless everybody's more important interests have first been seen to. If, for instance, people's need for health is more important than their aesthetic enjoyment, then those public authorities who allocate resources to the development of medical services are morally on a higher plane than political leaders who sponsor the arts while the citizens of the country suffer from curable ailments.[14]

Cases where the basic, or most important, interests or needs of individuals are in conflict are problematical in virtually all theories of justice. The version of liberalism that I subscribe to insists that, ideally, everybody's basic needs should be satisfied to the degree that this is compatible with the equal satisfaction of everybody else's basic needs. Factors like gender, age, social status and the colour of one's skin should not be taken into account in the assessment.

There are, however, certain exceptions to the principle of strict equality. If the conflict is caused by an individual who deliberately and without provocation tries to interfere with another person's basic need-satisfaction, then it is not necessary to give any consideration to the needs of the guilty party if they are in conflict with the victim's needs. Similarly, if it can be shown that industrious persons are in a better position than idle persons who initially had the same opportunities, then it is not right to reduce the basic need-satisfaction of the hard-working to assist the lazy. The catch here is, though, that it is very difficult to find groups or even individuals who have had exactly the same opportunities at any particular point in time. Yet another class of exceptions is formed by the cases where ascriptions of guilt and merit do not apply but where everybody's basic needs cannot, for lack of resources, be fully satisfied. Perfectly just decisions are in these cases impossible, but among the least unjust solutions are, I think, the use of lotteries and attempts to minimize the number of individuals whose needs cannot be satisfied.

If fully informed and reasonably autonomous persons freely decide to act in ways which can be harmful to themselves – but not to others – their actions should not, according to Mill's view, be forcibly restricted. It is acceptable that others warn them or try to persuade them, but the use of threats and physical force is precluded. The situation is, of course, different when it comes to persons who are not fully informed or reasonably autonomous, or whose choices are not freely made.

Temporary emotional disturbances and lack of knowledge provide good reasons for the limited use of force. If a person reacts to tragic news by trying to jump out of a tenth-floor window, it would not normally be wrong to seize her. And if another person is purposefully walking towards an extremely dangerous bridge, anybody can legitimately grab his hand to inform him about its condition. But in both cases the justification for the use of force is the agent's mental state, not the potential harm. When the person who heard the tragic news has calmed down, others are no longer entitled to hinder her actions. And when the information regarding the danger has been passed on to the pedestrian, he must be allowed to cross the bridge if he so chooses.

Individuals who are not capable of sufficiently autonomous decision-making can be legitimately protected from self-inflicted harm. Small children and persons who are senile or mentally ill cannot always make genuinely self-determined choices, and when this is the case, their freedom must not be respected if they are likely to cause themselves physical or psychological damage. The proper limits of the constraints on their liberty can be determined by estimating what their own autonomous choice would probably be if they were capable of self-determined thinking.

Similar principles can be applied to individuals who act under undue economic or social pressure. If, for instance, an individual decides to sell one of her kidneys in order to pay her debts, the decision is not necessarily immune to restrictions just because she is fully informed and reasonably autonomous in the psychological sense. The economic pressure she faces can be caused by other people's negligence or malevolence, in which case appeals to her individual liberty alone do not self-evidently justify the purchase of the vital organ. Duelling is an often cited example of similar pressures which are social or cultural rather than financial in nature.

According to the credos of Millian liberalism competent individuals are fully entitled to make choices which they themselves or others regard as irrational. Rationality and irrationality can be defined in many ways, but no morally neutral description can in and by itself legitimize the use of coercion or force against persons who act in defiance with reason but inflict no harm on others. Besides, most forms of rationality are such that individuals cannot even in theory be forced to assume them. The consistency and realism of people's beliefs, which is sometimes seen as a hallmark of rationality, can be increased by education but it can seldom be furthered by legal sanctions.

Some moralists have challenged this strictly liberal view by arguing that irrational decisions are never autonomous: individuals who continuously make them should be likened to the mentally ill and the emotionally disturbed. The proponents of more moderate doctrines have suggested, accordingly, that choices which are not rational should be restricted on the grounds that they are not sufficiently self-determined. But seen from the Millian viewpoint this argument is skewed. When competent human beings make informed decisions without the coercive influence of others, the ensuing actions are autonomous in the relevant technical sense even when they can also be depicted as self-destructive or silly.

The restriction of choices which are considered irrational have sometimes also been defended by claiming that they are immoral. The claim is, of course, valid in cases where other people would be harmed by the unreasoned exercise of freedom. But this is not what the critics of the Millian creed normally mean. Morality, or 'morality as such', is in their book not definable by the beneficial and harmful consequences of actions.

When harmless actions are called 'immoral as such', the ethical ideals underlying the locution can be classified either as deontological or as teleological. The deontological way of thinking can be further divided into the intellect-based and emotion-based approaches, and the teleological models into the theological and the secular.

For those who hold the intellect-based deontological view, the most important ethical consideration is the moral law as defined by human reason. Actions and policies are objectionable if they violate the absolute precepts of morality – for instance, the categorical imperative, the humanity principle, or certain rights which are regarded as absolute. The main problem of this view is that it is not easy to determine where, exactly, the limits set by the principles ought to be drawn. This is probably why very few philosophers have even tried to apply the model to questions in medicine and health care.[15]

For the proponents of emotion-based deontological thinking, feelings are the paramount concern of ethics. If we feel that certain actions or policies are bad, evil, disgusting, unnatural or immoral, they should be banned. One major difficulty with this model is that it is exceedingly relativistic. In most cases there is no consensus concerning our emotional responses, and many questions remain, therefore, unanswered. Whose feelings should be respected? Should actions be banned only if *everybody* feels that they are bad? Or is it sufficient that the *majority* feel that way? Or perhaps prohibitions ought to be employed if a significant *minority* nurtures these feelings? Or should we say that if *anybody* at all feels this way, the policies which provoke the reactions ought to be rejected?[16]

Those who hold the theological teleological view place their trust on the moral law as defined by the church or the clerics. If these religious authorities condemn some actions as unethical, they ought to be banned. The problem with this model in the present context is that although knowledge regarding different religious moralities can help us, in the sociological sense, explain people's attitudes towards issues in bioethics, theological views cannot, philosophically speaking, justify those attitudes.

For the proponents of the secular teleological view, the stress of ethics is on personal or social perfection. Medical procedures and health care provision should be condoned only if they are consistent with the *telos*, or the natural goal, of human beings in a just society. The two questions that the champions of this view ought to answer satisfactorily before they can claim universal recognition for their ideals are: 'What is the natural goal of human life, and who is to define it?' and 'When can we call a society just?'

Theorists who hold essentially deontological or teleological views, but who admit that it is not always easy to justify them, can argue that morality as such should be respected because conscientious individuals will otherwise be offended by the immorality of the liberal policies. This can mean two things. If it means that actual, unavoidable psychological harm will be inflicted on people who cannot change their views without considerable cost, then a weak prima facie justification for restrictions can be seen to emerge. But this is a justification founded on other-regarding harm, not on any other categorical rules. If, on the other hand, the offence in question is limited to the sore feelings of moralistic individuals, then the remarks concerning emotion-based thinking that I presented above apply.

The liberal dislike towards moralism has been seen by some of its critics as self-contradictory.[17] They argue that while liberalism is supposed to be a morally neutral theory, its proponents have turned it into a full-blown ethical doctrine which condemns, among other things, religious fundamentalism and political conservatism. The opponents take this to mean that the alleged advocates of liberty are, as a matter of fact, themselves champions of one type of moralism, namely liberal moralism.

This argument completely misses the point of liberal thinking. The Millian model does require people to act responsibly in matters which concern other people. But unlike religious fundamentalism and political conservatism it does not make any demands when it comes to choices which concern only individuals themselves. Therefore it is misleading to compare liberalism to the various forms of moralism which expect people's obedience both in the other-regarding and the self-regarding spheres of life. The common denominator of different types of moralism is a tendency towards totalitarianism, which is alien to the liberal political morality.

In a comparison between liberalism and totalitarianism, which is in the end the only relevant juxtaposition here, most reasonable people can see the advantages of the liberty-respecting alternative. Although individuals can primarily hope that the rules enforced by laws and social policies were the ones they themselves prefer, they must also see how badly they would fare if the rules were set by their fiercest opponents. A liberal system is – on the social and political level – the best, because it is – individually – the second best alternative to everybody.[18]

The normative approach that I have sketched in this chapter is intended to amalgamate all the good elements of Millian liberalism.[19] Compressed in the form of three concise principles, these are:

The principle of liberty   The liberty and autonomy of competent, well-informed, free agents must be fully respected and maximally protected in matters which concern only or mainly themselves.

The principle of equality   The needs and interests of all individuals ought to be taken equally into account in public decision-making.

The principle of responsibility   The responsibility of individuals for the welfare of their fellow beings should be enforced in matters where the choices of individuals concern the needs and interests of others.

These principles have, obviously, been applied to medical matters before, but all the previous attempts have, I think, tended to ignore at least one of them. The mid-level principlism of Tom Beauchamp and James Childress[20] and the liberalism of John Kleinig [21] leave room for moralistic attitudes in cases where the principle of responsibility could be more naturally employed. The positive utilitarianism of Peter Singer[22] and the negative utilitarianism of John Harris,[23] in their turn, sometimes seem to disregard the autonomy and integrity of individuals.

The originality of my approach, if any, is that in the following chapters I have tried to keep all three principles in my mind at all times. The principle of responsibility occupies perhaps the most prominent role in the life-and-death considerations of the first chapter, but the principles of liberty and equality gradually come to the fore when I turn my attention to slightly less dramatic issues.

Notes

1   This thesis has been developed further in H. Häyry and M. Häyry, 'Applied philosophy at the turn of the millennium', in O. Leaman (ed.), *The Future of Philosophy: Towards the 21st Century* (London and New York: Routledge, 1997).

2   See, e.g., G. Grisez and J.M. Boyle, *Life and Death with Liberty and Justice: A Contribution to the Euthanasia Debate* (Notre Dame, Ind.: University of Notre Dame Press, 1979); B. Häring, *The Law of Christ* (Westminster, Md.: Newman Press, 1966); D.H. Labby (ed.), *Life and Death: Ethics and Options* (Seattle, Wa.: University of Washington Press, 1968); J.T. Noonan Jr (ed.), *The Morality of Abortion: Legal and Historical Perspectives* (Cambridge, Mass: Harvard University Press, 1970).

3   On the first part of this view see, e.g., J. Harris, *The Value of Life* (London: Routledge & Kegan Paul, 1985); J. Harris, *Wonderwoman and Superman: The Ethics of Human Biotechnology* (Oxford and New York: Oxford University Press, 1992); H. Kuhse, *The Sanctity-of-Life Doctrine in Medicine: A Critique* (Oxford and New York: Oxford University Press, 1987); P. Singer, *Practical Ethics* (Cambridge: Cambridge University Press, 1979). On the second part of the view see, e.g., J. Feinberg, *Harm to Self* (Oxford and New York: Oxford University Press, 1986); H. Häyry, *The Limits of Medical Paternalism* (London and New York: Routledge, 1991).

4   On definitions of freedom see, e.g., J. Kleinig, *Paternalism* (Manchester: Manchester University Press, 1983), pp. 19–21.

5   W.A. Parent, 'Freedom as the non-restriction of options', *Mind* **83** (1974): 432–434; M. Häyry and T. Airaksinen, 'Hard and soft offers as constraints', *Philosophia* **18** (1988): 385–398. Cf. S.I. Benn and W.L. Weinstein, 'Being free to act, and being a free man', *Mind* **80** (1971): 194–211; S.I. Benn and W.L. Weinstein, 'Freedom as the non-restriction of options: A rejoinder', *Mind* **83** (1974): 435–438; H. Steiner, 'Individual liberty', *Proceedings of the Aristotelian Society* **75** (1974–75): 33–50; J.P. Day, 'Threats, offers, law, opinion and

liberty', *American Philosophical Quarterly* **14** (1977): 257–272; D. Miller, 'Constraints on freedom', *Ethics* **94** (1983): 66–86.

6   See J. Feinberg, *Social Philosophy* (Englewood Cliffs, NJ: Prentice-Hall, 1973), pp. 13–14.

7   Feinberg 1973, p. 13.

8   On 'positive' and 'negative' freedom see, e.g., I. Berlin, 'Two concepts of liberty' (originally appeared 1958), reprinted in his *Four Essays on Liberty* (Oxford: Oxford University Press, 1969); and C. Taylor, 'What's wrong with negative liberty?', in A. Ryan (ed.), *The Idea of Freedom* (Oxford: Oxford University Press, 1979).

9   J. Feinberg, *Rights, Justice, and the Bounds of Liberty* (Princeton: Princeton University Press, 1980), pp. 40 ff.; J. Feinberg, *Harm to Others* (Oxford and New York: Oxford University Press, 1984), p. 212; Kleinig 1983, p. 51.

10   The classical statement of this view is J.S. Mill, *On Liberty* (originally published 1859), reprinted in R. Wollheim (ed.), *Three Essays* (Oxford: Oxford University Press, 1975), pp. 22 ff.

11   Mill 1859, pp. 14–15.

12   See, e.g., H. Häyry and M. Häyry, 'Liberty, equality, utility – Classical to liberal utilitarianism', in T.D. Campbell (ed.), *Law and Enlightenment in Britain* (Aberdeen: Aberdeen University Press, 1990); M. Häyry, *Liberal Utilitarianism and Applied Ethics* (London and New York: Routledge, 1994).

13   See, e.g., J.S. Mill, *Utilitarianism* (first published 1861), reprinted in J.S. Mill and J. Bentham, *Utilitarianism and Other Essays*, ed. by A. Ryan (Harmondsworth, Middlesex: Penguin Books, 1987), pp. 335–338.

14   On the sacrifice of the minorities within utilitarian theories, see Häyry 1994, chapters 2 and 3.

15   Ruth Chadwick is an exception – see, e.g., her article 'The market for bodily parts: Kant and duties to oneself', *Journal of Applied Philosophy* **6** (1989): 129–139.

16   The only proper attempt to answer these questions is Patrick Devlin's 'Morals and the criminal law' (originally appeared 1959), reprinted in his *Enforcement of Morals* (Oxford and New York: Oxford University Press, 1965). But Devlin's vindication of intolerance and disgust has two flaws. First, it is philosophically

invalid (see, e.g., Häyry 1991, pp. 96-104). And second, it is almost certainly inapplicable to most issues in bioethics, as the woman or man in the street does not normally have sufficient knowledge concerning the arrangements of health care provision to assess in a reasonable manner 'whether, looking at it calmly and dispassionately, we regard it as a vice so abominable that its mere presence is an offence' (Devlin 1959, p. 17).

17   See, e.g., S. Lee, *Law and Morals* (Oxford and New York: Oxford University Press, 1986), pp. 15-17.

18   I have developed this argument in more detail in Häyry 1991, pp. 106-108.

19   This book is not intended to be an exercise in Mill scholarship, and I must emphasize that what I have said above is what *I think* Mill said in *On Liberty*. But even if he did not, it does not matter, because my formulation is in any case a possible interpretation of the kind of utilitarian liberalism that Mill tried to create.

20   T. Beauchamp and J. Childress, *Principles of Biomedical Ethics*, fourth edition (Oxford and New York: Oxford University Press, 1994).

21   Kleinig 1983.

22   Singer 1979.

23   Harris 1985.

1 Who is to Live and Who is to Die?

One of the most important and most difficult issues in bio-medical ethics today is that of killing people and letting them die. There are certain medical situations in which the killing or allowing to die of one human being is the only way to save the life and health of another human being. In the present chapter my purpose is to examine situations of that kind – to sketch out some model situations, to analyse them, and to find out whether there are any general rules to be employed in making decisions about them. As things are today, physicians are used to making life-and-death decisions according to their own conventional ideas about medical ethics. I whould like to show that at least in certain specific situations some other kinds of criteria could be used, instead.

False Criteria Employed by Medical Professionals

A hypothetical example will be useful for the purpose of making a few introductory remarks. Let us assume that we have two patients, both in serious trouble with their breathing, but only one machine to maintain their respiration artificially. The situation is presented schematically in Figure 1.1.

		Patient A	
		Lifesaving equipment used	Lifesaving equipment not used
Patient B	Lifesaving equipment used	IMPOSSIBLE!	POSSIBLE: Saves B and kills A
	Lifesaving equipment not used	POSSIBLE: Saves A and kills B	Possible but usually IRRATIONAL: Kills both A and B

Figure 1.1   The alternative courses of action

Equipped as we are with only one respirator it is impossible to choose the best alternative, that is, to save both patients. On the other hand, it would usually be irrational to choose the worst alternative, that is, not to save either one or the other, since one machine is, after all, available and it should (under any 'normal' circumstances) be utilized. Therefore, the best thing to do in a situation like this is to save the life of one patient even though it will very probably mean letting the other die. But the question, of course, is: Who is to live, and who is to die? Do we have any general rules for choices in these situations?

If the two patients in need of the same machine (e.g., a respirator) are similar to each other in all relevant respects, the only way to solve the problem may be to make a random decision, say, by tossing a coin. A random procedure is considered 'fair' because the same odds face every 'player' at the beginning. In real life, however, doctors seldom toss coins by the bedside. This is mainly because people differ from each other: the assumption of 'similarity in relevant respects' does not generally hold. But it is not at all clear, either, whether all the differences used by physicians to justify their decisions should really be regarded as relevant in our context. In what follows I shall present three obviously false views of 'relevant respects' in making life-and-death decisions.

Consider, for instance, a doctor who disconnects a patient, whom he or she does not know personally, from the respirator, and assigns the machine to a relative of his or hers, saying: 'Look, there is a difference between them! This one is my relative, my flesh and blood, but that one isn't.' There is obviously something morally dubious in this statement; it simply cannot be used by enlightened people. (The reason is, from a Kantian point of view, that the imperative implicit in the statement contains a particular individual term, 'I'. From a utilitarian point of view, the physician is wrong because nepotism does not necessarily lead to the best possible consequences in the field of social co-operation.)

Or another doctor could make use of the principle 'first come, first served', according to which the first patient in need of a machine gets it, and all others have to do without. But why should it be that the first to come should always be served first? Quite obviously, before the arrival of another patient, the first one may freely occupy the machine. But as soon as the second patient enters the picture, an independent decision should be made about the renewed priorities. And since in this novel situation both patients are equally present, there are no grounds for using the 'first come, first served' principle any more. Why not 'second come, second served': one patient has already had his or her share of the scarce medical aid available, now it is time to help the other? The principle 'first come, first served' cannot be used in medical decision-making since coming first (or second or third etc.) does not constitute a relevant difference between patients.

Still another doctor could refer to the words of Arthur Clough, the poet, who wrote:

Thou shalt not kill; but need'st not strive
Officiously to keep alive.[1]

The verse is usually supposed to defend a view according to which it may be right to let a human being die but it is always wrong to kill one. Some doctors think that terminating a patient's artificial respiratory aid means killing the patient, and therefore they may also think that the patient already connected to the machine (in this case the respirator) should stay connected. But this, in its turn, is a mere application of the principle 'first come, first served' which we have already found objectionable above. In sum, then, doctors facing life-and-death decisions can and probably do employ reasons that do not stand well systematic criticism.

Human Beings who are not yet Persons

There are, however, three very important and elementary grounds for making relevant distinctions, which often escape the attention of medical decision-makers, namely, (1) the fact that one of the patients is not yet a person, (2) the fact that one of the patients is no longer a person, and (3) the reflected and declared will of the patients themselves. I shall consider these factors one by one in the following three sections. I shall begin, in the present section, by examining the status of human fetuses as patients (in a sense), but not yet persons.

In some pregnancies the fetus can become stuck inside the woman in such a way that it cannot be removed from the womb without a craniotomy, that is, without crushing its skull. The only other possibility is to wait until the woman dies – her death will occur sooner or later if an abortion is not performed – and remove the fetus unharmed from her dead body afterwards.[2]

As in the respirator situation described above, it is impossible to save both patients, and irrational not to save either one or the other. Therefore, it is again clear in this situation that we ought to save one human being at the cost of the life of another human being. But which one should it be? The Roman Catholic Church suggests that since performing a craniotomy would kill the fetus while by taking no action one would only let the woman die, the decision should be made in favour of the fetus.[3] Unfortunately for women, the Roman Catholic Church is very influential in some parts of the world, and doctors really do make their decisions along the dictated lines.

From a philosophical point of view, however, there is not much to be said for this doctrine.[4] Consider, for instance, a young girl who has become pregnant through rape, and who would die if she gave birth to her aggressor's child. The doctors around her hospital bed say: 'We are so sorry not to be able to help you, but you see, we really aren't permitted to kill the fetus, and so we just have to let you die.' Situations like this seem quite inhumane, even absurd, and yet they are an indispensable corollary to holding the doctrine that killing and letting die are, morally speaking, always clearly separable.

What I have said above does not, however, solve the main problem, namely the choice between the two alternatives. Counterexamples like the one I have just presented may convince us that even if it were generally worse to kill a human being than to let a human being die, we could not rely on that principle in exceptional cases. But all that this proves is that fetuses shoud not be automatically preferred to pregnant women in their mutual struggle to stay alive. What remains to be seen is, do women possess any privileges over and above fetuses, or are the positions of the two groups (at least prima facie) equal. If the latter is the case, the rights and interests of both parties should be weighed equally, and we should return to our starting point, in other words, tossing the coin would be our best choice.[5] But there is another possible line of thinking. Perhaps different kinds of beings have different amounts of rights. It can be proposed, accordingly, that since fetuses are not yet actual persons (I shall return to the notion of a 'person' in the following section), their right to life is less weighty than the right to life of a woman.[6] Therefore, the woman should have priority in our case: the fetus should be killed to save the woman.

Unfortunately, however, it is not clear how much weight we can put on this suggestion. Utilitarians say that the names of various 'rights' are mere abbreviations for some complex interpersonal situations. We cannot, therefore, begin an ethical conversation with 'rights' - if they occur in that conversation at all, they must occur at the end.[7] Anti-utilitarians, on the other hand, may quite intelligibly claim that there are no degrees pertaining to rights: once I have attained the right to life, I really possess it - nobody is permitted to take my life away from me.[8] As we can see, the suggestion that rights could have degrees according to their relative weight is problematical, and thus we cannot necessarily rely on it.

Throughout the section hints have been made towards a possible solution to our craniotomy problem. If we compare a pregnant woman to a fetus, the difference is clear. On the one hand we usually have a full-fledged human being, a person with full human rights, on the other hand we have a mere sentient being with no expectations and no preferences yet, in a word, a merely potential person. If the fetus is not born, nobody will be harmed, since there is nobody to be harmed.[9] Some people seem to think that 'potentiality' entails a fully developed person, an adult human being with full rights and interests living somehow 'in' the fetus – like an enchanted prince in a frog in fairy tales.[10] As soon as we rid ourselves of this conception, we should be able to discern the right course of action from the wrong one in our example (as well as in any other abortion situation). Fetuses do not exist as persons yet, and therefore they do not have any rights or interests that need protecting or would justify letting a pregnant woman die. On the other hand, women do have rights and interests – among them, the right to life – which can and should be protected by performing the craniotomy. Thus the decision creates no difficulties, after all. Every time we have two patients, an actual person and a merely potential one, only one of whom can be saved, we should decide in favour of the actual person, in our example in favour of the woman. This, then, is the first general rule to be followed in some (seemingly) difficult life-and-death decisions.

Human Beings who are not Persons any More

Let us now turn to the second of my three suggested (and supposedly relevant) differences. What should we do, if we have a brain-dead patient connected to our only respirator while another, otherwise relatively healthy patient will soon die if he or she is not connected to the same respiratory device?

It would be once again impossible to save both patients, and once again irrational to let both of them die. But the apparent symmetry of the remaining two decision alternatives may this time well be challenged. In fact, the asymmetry is obvious once we call attention to what can and what cannot be said about the decisions. If we choose to disconnect the brain-dead patient in order to connect up the other one, we can be said to have saved the latter. Similarly, if we choose not to disconnect the brain-dead patient, we can be said to have let the other patient die. What cannot intelligibly be said, however, is that we could have killed the brain dead patient or saved him or her by disconnecting or not disconnecting the body from the respirator. The impossibility of these latter locutions is of a logical (or, conceptual) nature. How can somebody who is already dead be killed? And how can somebody who is already dead be saved (in a secular sense)? The only reason to use these expressions seems to be the false belief that brain dead human beings are not really dead. But they are, and that is what I shall attempt to show in the present section.

Traditionally death has been defined as the cessation of blood circulation, respiration, pulsation, and other essential animal and vital functions of the human body.[11] Only quite recently has the concept of brain death become central in bio-medical discussions of the human death. Besides, the urge for redefining death in terms of the stoppage of brain functions did not emerge from any theoretical considerations but from the rapidly increasing practice of organ transplantations. If the patient is defined to be alive as long as his or her heart beats, a heart transplantation would mean killing one patient to provide another one with a functioning heart. Or should we perhaps say that after the operation the donor is still alive since his or her heart still beats – albeit in a new body – while the patient with the new heart is dead since his or her heart does not beat any more? Certainly not, and this is where we bring in the notion of 'brain death' to sweep our conceptual difficulties under the carpet. A human being is brain dead if and only if the activity of his or her central nervous system has finally ceased.[12] And, according to reliable medical sources in several countries, brain-dead human beings are dead. Unfortunately, however, the brain dead themselves do not agree with the 'reliable medical sources', and – with a little mechanical help – they continue their biological living, that is, at least their bodies are still alive.[13] Brain-dead human beings are not necessarily totally dead.

Two kinds of 'human death' should be distinguished here. First, a human being is not *biologically* dead until his or her body is totally disintegrated in respect to its organic functions. Thus the brain dead are not (immediately) biologically dead, since it is 'only' their brain that does not work any more. But secondly, a human being is *personally* dead as soon as his or her person ceases to exist, and this may occur well before the biological death, or the final disintegration of the body as a living organism. (By a 'person' I now refer simply to that something we know as a particular person – whatever the features are that make it 'personally' recognizable to us.) Accordingly, a particular patient, say, Jill Jones is alive only if both the patient is alive (biologically) and the patient (i.e. the being in the hospital bed) is still Jill Jones (the person).[14] Now if the patient called Jill Jones is brain-dead, her brain has irreversibly ceased functioning. This, in turn, means that she will never talk again, walk again, be happy or sad again – in fact, she will never again experience anything or expect anything of her life in the future. Thus the person we have known as Jill Jones is gone forever. Imagine another brain transplanted in her body, say, that of John Smith. If anything will come out of this operation, we shall probably have John Smith, the person, somehow inhabiting the former body of the late Jill Jones.[15] But as soon as the patient Jill Jones is brain-dead she – as a person – is dead, and the human organism artificially kept alive in a hospital bed should be of no further interest to those who have known her as a person. We could, of course, given that we had unlimited medical resources, keep all brain-dead human bodies biologically alive as long as possible. But in the world of scarce resources we have to content ourselves with compromises.

To return to our case, then, we are now in the position to say what to do in situations like the one described above. In case we have two patients (two living entities of the species homo sapiens) and only one machine to maintain their bodily functions artificially, we should first try to find out whether both of them are alive as persons. If this is not the case, we should decide in favour of the person who is alive. Therefore, in our example we should disconnect the brain-dead patient and connect up the other one. The general rule seems to be that doctors should always prefer persons to not-yet-persons or no-longer-persons. Unfortunately, this is not always the case.

Human Beings who Want to die

The third and last of my suggested differences between the two patients is that of willingness to live and willingness to die. We can have two patients, only one of whom can be saved; they can both be living and rational persons, but it can be the case that one of them wants to live while the other one wants to die. Consider, for instance, a hundred-year-old patient dying in great pain of cancer, who is not expected to live more than a few days, perhaps weeks, and who has wished to die for a long time if only the physicians would let this happen. Let us presume that this patient occupies the only respirator in the hospital – and that this is the only hospital in this particular little town, which is a long way away from other towns or hospitals or respirators. Let us further presume that in that very same little town a ten-year-old child happens to inhale some poisonous gases and would need the respirator for a couple of days to survive.

As in the previous cases, saving both would be impossible, and killing both (or letting both die) would be irrational. But this time the asymmetry between the two remaining alternatives is more obvious than ever. This is not only the case as regards our ability to exclude a patient from consideration on extrinsic grounds, but also as regards the patient's own intrinsic willingness not to go on living. Let us reflect on the situation more closely.

My claim is that in our example the doctors should disconnect the patient who wishes to be disconnected, and give all the artificial respiratory aid to the other patient, the child. Moreover, my claim is that the doctors should do this because the older patient wishes to die, and not for any other reason. To be sure, the child is younger – it might well be the case that the young should always be preferred to the old. But such a principle does not hold. Suppose the hundred-year-old patient in our example were relatively healthy and perfectly happy and likely to live at least ten more meaningful years (after, say, a month's stay in the respirator). It is at once clear that his or her human rights would be seriously undermined were we to let him or her die merely because of old age. The same point can be looked at from another angle, too. Suppose both patients were, say, fifty years old. If the rest of the original description remained unchanged it seems to be clear that the prescription would still remain: Let the patient who wishes to die, die, and save the other! But physicians do not always recognize the principle. Why?

There are at least three possible arguments against the solution I have recommended – disconnecting the older patient in order to connect the younger on the ground that the former wants to die. Firstly, disconnecting the older patient can be regarded as killing that patient, and killing – as opposed to letting somebody die – could be regarded as always forbidden. I have already dealt with this argument in the previous sections, and shall not return to it. Secondly, some doctors might agree with the solution, but disagree with the line of argumentation. In their opinion, doctors are the only ones capable of making ultimate life-and-death decisions. They can perhaps take into account the fact that one of the patients wishes to die but they find themselves under no obligation to fulfil the patients wishes as such. The attitude these doctors present – 'medical paternalism' – is without doubt well-grounded as far as ordinary medical treatment is concerned. We should take the prescribed amounts of medicine although it may taste terrible and we do not want to take it, and we should visit the dentist regularly although he or she may subject us to painful drilling we would like to avoid. But to be justified, medical paternalism must serve a purpose: it must be aimed at the good of the patients. If the patient really wants to die, dying would probably be the best thing for him or her, and thus medical paternalism does not give valid reasons for keeping him or her alive. The question, of course, is whether anybody can rationally wish to die, and whether we can ever know it. This brings us to the third argument against my solution.

Medical paternalism is, it can be argued, justified in our case because no rational human being wants to die. Survival is the basic concern of every human being: everybody wants to continue living, to experience more, to see what the world will give tomorrow. All this is quite plausible, I think, but only in ordinary life. Our hundred-year-old patient was described as being in great pain, and was not expected to live long anyway. His or her decision is not a matter of choosing between living or dying, but between dying quietly now or dying very painfully after a few more days' or weeks' suffering. The difference is obvious, and I think it is also obvious that people can rationally wish to die in circumstances like these. The other side of the problem remains, however. Can we ever know reliably that a human being wants to die? People change their minds, and we could by accident kill somebody who does not really want to die, although he or she could apparently want it. Admittedly, we have a difficulty here. But I find it important to observe that the difficulty is a factual, not a conceptual one. It may be difficult to know what a human being wants, but it is not impossible. And once we know that the older patient in our example wants to die, we should disconnect him or her in order to connect the younger patient. The considered will of the patient is one of the relevant factors in difficult life-and-death decisions. I shall return to this question in more detail in chapter 2.

Other Alternatives

We have now found three general selective rules for difficult medical two-person choices. Whenever we are faced with the situation of having two patients, only one of whom can be saved, we should always prefer persons to not-yet-persons and no-longer-persons, and take into account the patient's wish to die. There may be other similarly obvious rules to be employed as well, but I shall content myself with these in the present context.[16] I shall conclude my examination by making a couple of remarks about the non-discussed squares of my schematic figure.

In the figure presented at the outset of this chapter I mentioned that it would usually be irrational to let both of the patients die. The qualification 'usually' derives from the considerations in the preceding section. We could have two patients, both wishing to die rather than to live. In such situations it would probably not be irrational or forbidden to let both of them die. I shall not, however, go into presenting arguments in favour of my intuitive inclination, since that would lead us straight into the very difficult problems of euthanasia, which will be dealt with in the following chapter. Instead, I shall say a few words about the remaining square of our figure.

Let us assume that the only relevant rules in these situations are the ones I have presented. Since the two patients can both be persons and since persons usually want to live, the only solution in most cases will be something like tossing the coin. But – fair or not – the thought of doctors organizing hospital lotteries in order to decide who is to live and who is to die seems rather absurd. Some of these undesirable lotteries can be avoided, however. The impossibility of saving both patients is often due to a lack of material resources. Therefore, many situations can be solved in advance by buying the right machines for the right places. But when this is not possible, general rules are needed for ultimate medical decision-making. The three rules put forward in the present paper are perhaps the most obvious ones to be taken into account.

Notes

An earlier version of this chapter has been published as Heta Häyry, 'Who is to live and who is to die? A study on some ultimate medical decisions', *Praxiology* **4-5** (1990): 85-97. My thanks are due to Timo Airaksinen and Matti Häyry for their helpful comments, and to Dr Mark Shackleton, Lecturer in English, University of Helsinki, for checking my English.

1 Cited in Peter Singer's *Practical Ethics* (Cambridge University Press, 1979), p. 149. Singer notes (p. 229), that the entire poem can be found in *The New Oxford Book of English Verse* (Oxford, 1978) edited by Helen Gardner.

2 See, e.g., Jonathan Bennett's article 'Whatever the consequences' in J. Rachels (ed.), *Moral Problems: A Collection of Philosophical Essays* (New York: Harper & Row, 1971).

3 On this widely discussed question of killing fetuses 'unlawfully' see, e.g., Philippa Foot's 'The problem of abortion and the doctrine of the double effect' in Rachels 1971; Daniel Callahan's *Abortion: Law, Choice and Morality* (London: The Macmillan Company, 1970), ch. 12; John T. Noonan Jr.'s 'An almost absolute value in history' in J.T. Noonan (ed.), *The Morality of Abortion. Legal and Historical Perspectives* (Cambridge, Mass.: Harvard University Press, 1970); Eike-Henner W. Kluge's *The Practice of Death* (New Haven and London: Yale University Press, 1975), p. 62 ff.; Alan Donagan's *The Theory of Morality* (Chicago and London: The University of Chicago Press, 1979), pp. 157-164); Philip E. Devine's *The Ethics of Homicide* (Ithaca and London: Cornell University Press, 1978), ch. 4; and Germain Grisez and Joseph M. Boyle Jr.'s *Life and Death with Liberty and Justice. A Contribution to the Euthanasia Debate* (Notre Dame: University of Notre Dame Press, 1979).

4 Thoroughly shown in Bennett 1971. See also Judith Jarvis Thomson's 'A defence of abortion' in *Philosophy and Public Affairs* **1** (1971): 47-66; Michael Tooley's 'Abortion and infanticide' in *Philosophy and Public Affairs* **2** (1972): 37-65; and Jonathan Glover's *Causing Death and Saving Lives* (Harmondsworth, Middlesex: Penguin Books, 1977), ch. 7.

5   See, e.g., Germain Grisez's *Abortion: the Myths, the Realities, and the Arguments* (New York: Corpus Books, 1970), p. 94; and Baruch Brody's 'Thomson on abortion' in *Philosophy and Public Affairs* 1 (1972): 335-340.

6   This view has been presented by Alan Gewirth in *Reason and Morality* (Chicago: The University of Chicago Press, 1978), pp. 105, 121-122, 142-144, and Norman C. Gillespie in his article 'Abortion and human rights' in *Ethics* 87 (1976-1977): 237-243.

7   See e.g. Richard Brandt's 'The concept of a moral right and its function' in the *Journal of Philosophy* **LXXX** (1983): 29-45.

8   A certain view of the absoluteness of a 'right' is included, e.g., in Ronald Dworkin's *Taking Rights Seriously* (London: Duckworth, 1977), esp. pp. 91-92.

9   On interests, harms, and their relevance for the present subject see, e.g., Tooley 1972; R.M. Hare, 'Abortion and the Golden Rule' in *Philosophy and Public Affairs* 4 (1975): 201-222; M. Bayles, 'Harm to the unconceived' in *Philosophy and Public Affairs* 5 (1976): 292-304; Singer 1979, chs 4 and 6; and A.R. White, *Rights* (Oxford: Clarendon Press, 1984), ch. 6.

10 An analogy beautifully developed in Robert M. Gordon's article 'The abortion issue' in R. Freeman (ed.), *The Abdication of Philosophy. Philosophy and the Public Good* (La Salle, Ill.: Open Court, 1976).

11 The factual knowledge about death I utilize in this section derives mainly from Finnish sources. The *Finnish Medical Journal* published in 1979 various articles on brain death (*Suomen Lääkärilehti - Finlands läkartidning* 13/79: 1042-1053). 'Elämä ja kuolema' ('Life and death') by Kalle Achté, Lauri Autio and Tapani Tammisto in K. Achté et al. (eds), *Lääkintäetiikka* (*Medical Ethics*) (Vaasa: Suomen Lääkäriliitto, 1982) includes a clear description of 'traditional' and brain death criteria. See also *A Definition of Irreversible Coma. Report of the Ad Hoc Committee of the Harvard Medical School to Examine the Definition of Brain Death*, reprinted e.g. in J.A. Behnke and S. Bok (eds), *The Dilemmas of Euthanasia* (Garden City, N.Y.: Anchor Press/Doubleday, 1975). The philosophical and ethical problems of the definitions of death are interestingly illuminated in Lawrence C. Becker's 'Human being: The boundaries of the concept' in *Philosophy and Public Affairs* 4 (1975): 334-359; David Lamb's 'Diagnosing death' in *Philosophy and Public Affairs* 7 (1978): 144-155; and Michael B. Green's and Daniel Wikler's 'Brain death and personal identity' in *Philosophy and Public Affairs* 9 (1980): 105-133.

12 This definition by *Webster's Ninth New Collegiate Dictionary* (Springfield, Mass.: Merriam-Webster, 1983) is as good as any definition of brain death.

There is a difference of opinions as to whether a mere 'upper' brain cessation of functioning qualifies as brain death or do we have to wait until the whole brain (including the 'lower' brain) is dead. When the 'morally relevant death' is defined as the disappearance of the person – see below – the irreversible coma (or, the final cessation of 'upper' brain functions) is quite sufficient in defining death. (See Green and Wikler 1980) I shall use the word 'brain death' in a broad sense to include 'upper' as well as 'lower' brain death, although this is contrary to what (at least Finnish) physicians think to be a satisfactory definition.

13   See Green and Wikler 1980, pp. 106–114.

14   The story of Jones and Smith originates from Green and Wikler 1980, pp. 117–128.

15   Green and Wikler 1980, pp. 117–128.

16   For a good discussion about life-and-death choices as well as about medical ethics in general, see J. Harris, *The Value of Life. An Introduction to Medical Ethics* (London: Routledge & Kegan Paul, 1985).

2 Voluntary Euthanasia and Medical Paternalism

Rapid medical development has, during the twentieth century, made it possible for us to prolong human life well beyond the limit of what of our great grandparents would have considered to be the 'natural' end of life. There is nothing wrong with this development in itself, of course, but sometimes an observer may get the impression that the professional, or moral, codes of today's physicians have not yet reached the level that today's medical possibilities require. Doctors are still trying, in a Hippocratic spirit, to preserve human life whenever possible, despite the growing suspicion concerning the quality, or value, of the life they are 'protecting'.

The medical means that are used in maintaining bodily functions are not always pleasant for the patient. The patient may suffer and sometimes even say that he or she wishes to die rather than continue living under such conditions. But physicians, holding on to their life-preserving code, can answer the patient by saying either,

> (i)   'You don't really wish to to die!'

or

> (ii) 'You may, of course, really wish to die, but I cannot be sure of that!'

or

> (iii) 'You may really wish to die, and perhaps I can be reasonably sure of it, but your wish is irrational!'

All these statements are, of course, intended to justify the inevitable next line,

> (iv) 'Too bad you have to suffer, but I cannot let you die – let alone kill you.'

Statements (i–iii) express, I believe, the core of the medical paternalism physicians often use to reject voluntary euthanasia. But they also serve as the starting point and basis of my present attempt to show that any reasonably acceptable form of paternalism is compatible with fulfilling people's wishes when they really want to die. I shall first clarify what is usually meant by 'paternalism' and what forms it is supposed to take. I shall then go on to define 'euthanasia' and 'voluntary euthanasia'. After these considerations we should be in the position to study with some accuracy whether statements (i–iii) can be used to justify statement (iv) or not.

A Preliminary Definition of Paternalism

Paternalism can be (roughly) characterized as the attitude that people's own wishes should not always be respected since people do not or cannot always know what is good for them.[1] (The varieties of medical paternalism as well as other related attitudes and practices are examined more thoroughly in chapter 3.) The general idea underlying the attitude is that the 'good of man' is something objectively given and sometimes contrary to people's wishes and whims. This point is not necessarily a valid one. It could also be the case that people's own wishes and what is good for them cannot be separated at all – this is, at least, the credo of the liberal tradition. But even liberals have to admit that people do not always know what course of action is good for them in a particular situation, for the obvious reason that people do not always know what they ought to know, and cannot always use their knowledge in a proper manner. Their information concerning the situation they are in may be inadequate, or there may be something wrong with their reasoning.[2] Thus, at least sometimes, people's real wishes must be protected from their apparent ones.

   Two kinds of paternalism should be distinguished here.[3] The weak paternalism of the liberal doctrine is based on the conviction that people do usually know what is good for them, since what they wish – or 'really want' – is good for them. The only justified form of paternalism, according to this view, aims at ascertaining that people know what they are doing. The classical example of acceptable paternalistic interference within the liberal framework comes from J.S. Mill, who writes:

> If either a public officer or anyone else saw a person attempting to cross a bridge which had been ascertained to be unsafe, and there were no time to warn him of his danger, they might seize him and turn him back, without any real infringement of his liberty; for liberty consists in doing what one desires, and he does not desire to fall into the river.[4]

In Mill's example the man approaching the bridge does not seem to know what he is doing, that is, does not seem to notice that he is endangering himself. It is precisely this seeming lack of knowledge that justifies the interference. But, of course, it is also possible that the man is perfectly aware of the risk he is taking. He may know about the condition of the bridge, and he may realize the danger, and yet he may want to cross the bridge. In this case weak paternalism does not justify any further interference: once the man has expressed that it is his firm wish and intention to endanger himself by crossing the bridge regardless of its state, there is nothing more to be done.

Strong Paternalism

Weak paternalism is perhaps not a genuine kind of paternalism at all, for it is designed only to protect people's real wishes against their temporary ignorance or mental instability. Strong paternalism does not stop there. It states that, whatever people's wishes are and however informed and well-thought-out they seem to be, there is no decisive reason to respect them if it is not good for the people themselves. For instance, the man trying to cross the bridge in Mill's example is endangering himself, that is, risking harm to himself, and doing that is probably not good for him. Therefore an advocate of strong paternalism might consider him or herself justified in 'seizing him and turning him back' regardless of his own wishes. Only 'might consider', since naturally the paternalist also acknowledges some risks to be worth taking. Let us suppose, however, that the man is trying to cross the bridge just for fun, and that the odds are, say, five to one in favour of his falling into the river and drowning. What would a 'strong' paternalist say to justify his or her intervention?

Imagine that the following conversation takes place between the paternalist (A) and the person approaching the bridge (B):

A: Hey there! You can't cross the bridge now!
B: Why not?
A: Because it's not safe. You might fall into the river and drown.
B: I know that. So what?
A: You don't want to fall into the river and drown, do you?
B: Why not?
A: You don't want to die, do you?
B: Why not?

A (to him or herself):

> The man's a lunatic. I'll have to knock him out to keep him away from the bridge. (Knocks him out.) He'll thank me for this once he's well again.

I believe that this is roughly the way the 'strong' paternalist thinks. Anybody who does not seem to appreciate the basic values of human life, for instance, the continuation of life itself, must be irrational, or insane. The point has an apparent similarity to the weak form of paternalism: it seems to be open to the interpretation that there is a temporary defect in the person's reasoning processes, and once the defect is eliminated, he may again act according to his own wishes. But this is not the case. The 'defect' in the person's reasoning cannot be eliminated without eliminating, at the same time, his relevant wishes. The 'weak' paternalist considers the (in)capability of making decisions and the wish to die to be two distinct and mutually independent things. The 'strong' paternalist, on the other hand, does not make such a distinction between irrationality and the wish to die: for him, the wish to die is a sign, or a criterion, of irrationality. Accordingly, he or she cannot accept that anybody who wishes to die could be rational.

The 'strong' paternalist's reasoning obviously moves in circles here. Nevertheless, he or she may be right. We do have a certain conception of sane and rational human behaviour, and playing Russian roulette with five bullets just for fun is perhaps not a part of this conception. (The odds in crossing the bridge and falling, five to one, are the same as in playing Russian roulette with only one empty chamber.) It seems to be the case that behavioural signs of irrationality may perhaps be legitimately subjected to strong paternalistic intervention. But moreover, it seems to me – although I shall make no attempt to prove my contention at this stage – that behavioural signs of irrationality are the only even seemingly legitimate indications for resorting to strong paternalism. Thus, the important question is, 'What do we regard as signs of irrationality?' Or rather, to narrow the scope, 'Do we regard a certain suggested type of behaviour, such as crossing an unsafe bridge for fun, as a sign of irrationality?' I shall leave the question of crossing the bridge unanswered for the moment – I shall return to it after defining 'euthanasia', 'voluntary euthanasia' and 'voluntary medical euthanasia'. These definitions are needed to move forward in my argument.

What is Voluntary Medical Euthanasia?

Euthanasia means, literally, 'good death' or 'easy death'. I take it that 'good' and 'easy' are in this context two different things, both of which should be taken into account in defining the concept.[5] 'Easy death' only implies that somebody's death is caused in a gentle manner, so that he or she does not suffer: if this were the sole criterion for euthanasia, many gentle murderers would have to be called experts in euthanasia. But death is hardly 'good' for the person about-to-be murdered, if he or she is healthy and happy and wishes to live. Therefore, a characterization of the desirability of death should be included in the definition. Accordingly, by euthanasia I mean a death which is as easy and painless as possible and which is good for the dying person, that is, more desirable, from his or her own point of view, than continuing to live.

One step toward finding out whether or not death is a good thing for the dying person may be to ask the person herself whether she wants to live or die. Euthanasia can be divided into three categories according to three different answers to this question.[6] An answer in favour of living means that euthanasia is involuntary – if there is such a thing. (The concept of 'a good death which is against the wishes of the dying' comes quite close to being a contradiction in terms: in fact, within the liberal framework it *is* a contradiction in terms.) If, on the other hand, the dying person is not capable of forming or expressing opinions about her own life and death, only nonvoluntary euthanasia can take place. Finally, if the answer is in favour of dying, voluntary euthanasia is possible.

Since depressed and suffering people may utter many things that they will regret later, the mere words, 'I wish to die!' are not a sufficient sign of what the person really wants. Seeming voluntariness to die is no warrant either of the voluntariness of the victim or of the goodness of the death. This is why I think that it is out of place even to use the word 'euthanasia' in talking about the 'mercy killings' that people sometimes commit in exceptional situations, such as, say, when a badly wounded soldier must otherwise be left behind in the hands of (supposedly) cruel enemies. In these situations the magic words, 'I wish to die!' may have been uttered by the victim, but the killing itself is more likely to be the result of the killer's emotional and irrational response to the distress of a comrade than the conclusion of a rational inference concerning the good of the dying. In fact, perhaps the only environment in which one can talk properly about euthanasia is a well-equipped hospital. I shall confine my attention for the rest of this chapter to medical euthanasia, that is, to euthanasia in medically controlled situations.

By voluntary medical euthanasia I mean a good and easy death (in the above sense) brought about, after careful consideration, by medically competent personnel on the demand and because of the demand of the patients themselves. Let me specify this definition by a couple of remarks. First, although I have been using the term 'dying person', I do not wish to restrict the procuring of voluntary medical euthanasia to terminally ill patients. Sometimes euthanasia is needed exactly because 'natural' death seems to be so far away. This is why no reference to terminal illness is made in the definition. And secondly, I take it that the 'careful consideration' undertaken by the medical personnel concerns only one thing, namely, whether the patient really wants to die or not. The underlying assumption is that if the patient 'really wants to die', that is, if his or her free (uncoerced) decision to die is based on reliable information and is the result of rational, calm and careful deliberation, then it is, eo ipso, good for the patient to die.

Weak Paternalism and Voluntary Medical Euthanasia

Let us now turn to the statements introduced in the beginning of the paper. Suppose a patient says to a doctor, 'I wish to die!' and the doctor replies,

(i)   'You don't really wish to die!'

or

(ii)   'You may, of course, really wish to die, but I cannot be sure of that!'

and, consequently,

(iv)   'Too bad you have to suffer, but I cannot let you die – let alone kill you!'

What kind of medical paternalism is reflected in the doctor's answers? I do not think that the use of statements (i) or (ii) to justify (iv) necessarily reflects more than a weak paternalistic attitude towards the patient's wishes. In the first statement the doctor seems to be only calming down a patient who is in pain and does not know what he is saying – a clear case of the patient having temporary defects in receiving and handling information concerning the situation. In regard to the second statement the situation seems to be slightly different. Obviously the patient is quite calm already and has been trying to give reasons for the wish to die. The doctor's answer shows that she is standing on the borderline between weak and strong paternalism: either she has to admit that it is, at least in principle, possible to be sufficiently sure of the patient's wishes; or she must adopt the strong paternalistic attitude. (More about the latter solution in the following section.)

Weak medical paternalism is fully compatible with voluntary medical euthanasia. By definition, voluntary medical euthanasia can only take place if the patient has freely decided to die, and if the decision is based on reliable information and careful deliberation. Weak paternalism, in its turn, aims at protecting people's real wishes against their apparent ones, when the two differ from each other. But in the case of voluntary medical euthanasia the doctors can be reasonably sure about the patient's real wishes, and, therefore, weak paternalism offers no justification for further intervention. ('Intervention' must be taken here to mean either positive interference, i.e. keeping the patient alive against his wishes; or negative interference, i.e. not aiding the patient to die peacefully. The former constitutes a case of refusing passive euthanasia, the latter a case of refusing active euthanasia.)[7]

But suppose a doctor says that she can never be 'reasonably sure' about the patient's wish to die. The thing we should ask her, as a rejoinder, is whether she thinks she can ever be reasonably sure of anything. For instance, can she ever be reasonably sure about the patient's desire to live? If she says she cannot, how can she ever do anything either to keep the patient alive, or to kill him? The most obvious answer is, of course, that physicians always work for the good of their patients, whether they happen to know what the patients want or not. And it is supposed that it is good for every human being to live. But with this reply we enter the region of strong medical paternalism.

Strong Paternalism and Voluntary Medical Euthanasia

Statement (iii), introduced in the beginning of the chapter, is a 'strong' paternalist's answer to the patient's wish to die:

(iii)   'You may really wish to die, and perhaps I can be reasonably sure of it, but your wish is irrational!'

Let me first show how statement (iii) is probably expected to connect with the view that doctors keep working for the good of their patients irrespective of the latter's wishes. The supposed connection is very simple and can be stated in the form of an argument as follows:

(1)   It is good for every human being to live.
(2)   Dead human beings do not live.
(3)   Thus, it is bad for any human being to be dead.

(4)   Moreover, it is irrational to wish anything bad for oneself.

(5)   Therefore, it is irrational for any human being to wish to to be dead.

Some people might think that the conclusion (5) does not prove anything, since there is no reason whatsoever not to fulfil people's irrational wishes as well as their rational ones. Let us return, at this point, to Mill's bridge to see what can be wrong with this suggestion.

Suppose the man who attempts to cross the unsafe bridge in Mill's example does not give any reasons for his deed, except that he thinks it is fun to do dangerous things. Suppose, further, that the only access to the bridge is through a tightly controlled gate. How many of us would like to open the gate to somebody who says that he wants to risk his life for fun? Not very many, I suppose. We do make the distinction between rational and irrational wishes, and we do not always feel obliged to fulfil other people's clearly irrational wishes. We may be wrong in not feeling obliged to do so, but this is the way we sometimes think. This is also why there is at least some initial plausibility in the view that if it is irrational to wish to be dead, then voluntary medical euthanasia need not necessarily be accepted.

But what about the soundness of the argument? Does the conclusion (5) follow from the premises (1, 2 and 4)? I think it does not. The only thing we can conclude from premises 1 and 2, even if they are assumed to be true, is that those who are dead lack the good of being alive. It does not follow, however, that it is bad to be dead, since 'not good' does not necessarily imply 'bad'. Nothing positively bad follows from the lack of good. In this sense, the first conclusion (3) is false, and the rest of the argument evaporates with it.

There is a further objection to the formulation of the third statement (3) in the argument. If we apply the universal statement to a specific person, John Smith, what we get is this:

(3')   It is bad for John Smith to be dead.

But the sentence does not make sense. If John Smith is dead, he does not exist any more. How, then, could it be bad for him to be dead? The point is that the subject needed for the sentence always disappears immediately as the predicate becomes applicable to it. Strictly speaking, the sentence is self-contradictory.[8]

The 'strong' paternalist cannot justify paternalistic interventions with an invalid argument. But the argument can be reformulated to meet the objections that I have presented. Only the first premise (1) has to be saved:

the rest of the argument (2 to 4) is subject to any changes needed. The following reformulation escapes the previous errors:

(1)   It is good for every human being to live.
(6)   Death is the end of life.
(7)   Thus, death puts an end to something that is good for the dying person.
(8)   It is irrational to wish an end to anything that is good for oneself.
(9)   Therefore, it is irrational for any human being to wish to die.

I am not sure whether (8) is as convincing as (4) in the earlier formulation. But if we let that pass, it seems that if the first premise (1) holds, the whole argument will also hold. To be formally valid, it should be specified, of course, but we need not go into that here. Let us, instead, turn our attention to the first premise.

Is it Good for Every Human Being to Live?

According to the argument (1 to 9) it is irrational to wish to die, but only if it is good for every human being to live. The 'strong' paternalist assumes that it is, and it must be admitted that life is usually a good thing for a human being. But is it always? Philippa Foot has challenged this view in her essay 'Euthanasia'. I quote some paragraphs from the essay to present her way of thinking about the matter. Foot gives examples of prisoners and of severely handicapped and senile patients who seem to have very few, if any, reasons for living. She continues:

> It seems, therefore, that merely being alive even without suffering is not a good. [...] The idea we need seems to be that of life which is ordinary human life in the following respect – that it contains a minimum of basic human goods. What is ordinary in human life [...] is that a man is not driven to work far beyond his capacity; that he has the support of a family or community; that he can more or less satisfy his hunger; that he has hopes for the future; that he can lie down to rest at night. [...] Disease too can so take over a man's life that the normal human goods disappear. When a patient is so overwhelmed by pain or nausea that he cannot eat with pleasure, if he can eat at all, and is out of the reach of even the most loving voice, he no longer has ordinary human life in the sense in which the words are used here. And [...] crippling depression can destroy the enjoyment of ordinary goods as effectively as external circumstances can remove them.

The suggested solution is, then, that there is a certain conceptual connexion between life and good in the case of human beings. [...] However, it is not the mere state of being alive that can [...] itself count as a good, but rather life coming up to some standard of normality.[9]

In these paragraphs Foot gives us the key to our present problem. It is only ordinary human life, in Foot's sense, that is always good. Since everybody does not have such a life, it is not the case that 'it is good for every human being to live'.

With Foot's help we can now distinguish between the man on the bridge in Mill's example and the patient who asks for euthanasia. The man on the bridge is supposed to have a perfectly normal life; he is healthy; he has nothing to gain from risking his life. We have every reason to believe that his death would put an end to something that is of value to him. If he, nevertheless, insists on endangering himself by crossing the bridge just for fun, we quite naturally come to think that he lacks some important faculty of a sane human mind. Therefore, paternalistic intervention may seem to be justified, 'for his sake'. But voluntary medical euthanasia is an entirely different thing. The patient may have a miserable life; she may be in constant pain; she may have nothing to gain from the days or weeks or months or years she is supposed to live. Her death does not put an end to anything that would be of value to her. If from such premises the patient infers that she wishes to die, there is no reason in the world to call her wish irrational. Life simply is not always good, and in the cases it is not, paternalistic interventions cannot be justified even by a moderately interpreted strong paternalism.

A Strict Interpretation of Strong Paternalism

Some paternalists do, however, reject voluntary medical euthanasia. Their strict version of strong paternalism is based on the Moral Law or the Will of God. Perhaps it is not irrational to wish to die, they say, but it is immoral, or against God's will. People can rationally wish to die, but they ought not to.

Fortunately, we need not waste much time in this context to show what is wrong with the strict version of strong paternalism. Its main deficiency is obvious: it is not a form of genuine paternalism at all. If it is rational for Jill Jones to wish to die, we cannot keep her alive for her own good. We can keep her alive for the sake of the moral law, of course, or to fulfil God's demands, but the good of Jill Jones does not necessarily depend on these things. The only genuine forms of paternalism are the weak and moderately interpreted strong forms presented above.

Conclusions

In sum, then. Medical paternalism means, in practice, action or inaction for the good of the patients, but, at the same time, against their own apparent or real wishes. 'Weak' paternalists finds it acceptable to protect people's real wishes from their apparent ones, while 'strong' paternalists also sometimes find it acceptable to protect people from their real, but irrational, wishes. Voluntary medical euthanasia rules out, by definition, interventions based on the weak form of paternalism, since it can only take place when the patient really wishes to die. But, what may be more surprising, a reasonable interpretation of strong paternalism also justifies voluntary medical euthanasia. Thus, there is no acceptable way open to the doctors to reject requests for a good and easy death by referring to 'the good of the patient'.

Notes

An earlier version of this chapter has been published as Heta Häyry, 'Voluntary euthanasia and medical paternalism', T. Airaksinen and W.W. Gasparski (eds), *Practical Philosophy and Action Theory* (New Brunswick and London: Transaction Publishers, 1993): 49-60. My thanks are due to Dr Mark Shackleton, Lecturer in English, University of Helsinki, for checking my English.

1   For a fuller characterization, see, e.g., J. Harris, *The Value of Life* (London: Routledge & Kegan Paul, 1985), pp. 192 ff.

2   See Harris 1985, pp. 195-200, on different kinds of 'defects' that can diminish a person's autonomy.

3   My discussion on the two kinds of paternalism draws a great deal from Joel Feinberg's 'Legal Paternalism', reprinted in his *Social Philosophy* (Englewood Cliffs, N.J.: Prentice-Hall, 1973): 45-52.

4   J.S. Mill, *On Liberty* (New York: Liberal Arts Press, 1956), p. 117. Cited in Feinberg 1973, p. 49.

5   For various definitions of euthanasia, see, e.g., E.-H.W. Kluge, *The Practice of Death* (London: Yale University Press, 1975), p. 173; P. Foot, 'Euthanasia', reprinted in her *Virtues and Vices* (Berkeley and Los Angeles: University of California Press, 1981), pp. 34-35; J. Glover, *Causing Death and Saving Lives* (Harmondsworth, Middlesex: Penguin Books, 1977), p. 182; S. Bok, 'Euthanasia

and care of the dying' in J.A. Behnke and S. Bok (eds), *The Dilemmas of Euthanasia* (Garden City, N.Y.: Anchor Press/Doubleday, 1975), pp. 1-4.

6   On divisions of euthanasia according to the patient's will, see, e.g., P.E. Devine, *The Ethics of Homicide* (London: Cornell University Press, 1978), p. 168; J. Fletcher, 'Infanticide and the ethics of loving concern' in M. Kohl (ed.), *Infanticide and the Value of Life* (Buffalo, N.Y.: Prometheus Books, 1978), p. 14; Foot 1981, pp. 51-55; Glover 1977, pp. 182, 191; G. Grisez and J.M. Boyle, *Life and Death with Liberty and Justice: A Contribution to the Euthanasia Debate* (Notre Dame, Ind.: University of Notre Dame Press, 1979), pp. 86-87; B. Russell, 'Still a live issue', *Philosophy and Public Affairs* **7** (1978): 278-281, p. 278; O. Russell, *Freedom to Die* (New York: Human Sciences Press, 1975), pp. 19, 21; P. Singer, *Practical Ethics* (Cambridge: Cambridge University Press, 1979), pp. 128-130.

7   On the differences and (moral) similarities between active and passive euthanasia, see, e.g., Foot 1981, pp. 48-51; Grisez and Boyle 1979, pp. 86-87; O. Russell 1975, pp. 19-20; Singer 1979, pp. 147-153.

8   See T. Nagel, 'Death', and M. Mothersill, 'Death', both in J. Rachels (ed.), *Moral Problems. A Collection of Philosophical Essays* (New York: Harper & Row, 1971).

9   Foot 1981, pp. 42-43.

3 Wrongful Medical Authoritarianism

One of the focal requirements of professional medical ethics is that physicians and nurses should under all circumstances regard their patient's best interest as paramount. This requirement implies, in fact, several principles, some of which are more controversial than others. Nobody would presumably deny that the patient's interests should be protected against natural forces such as diseases and injuries. Widespread agreement probably also prevails on the belief that patients should be protected against the unethical professional conduct of malevolent or negligent doctors and nurses. When it comes to social issues like protecting individual patients against the greater interests of the rest of society, disagreements are more likely to emerge. Not many people in the West believe in torturing political prisoners by using the latest medical technologies, but quite a few of us do believe in, say, quarantining people who carry fatal contagious diseases. In both cases the conflict occurs between the individual's rights and the general welfare of society.

One of the most vital controversies of health care ethics concerns, however, the protection of people's interests against their own expressed desires. Medical professionals often tend to think that their greater knowledge, experience and skills justify interventions which clash with the patient's prevailing preferences, granted that these interventions are expected to benefit the patient in the future. This opinion is by no means universally shared in modern societies.[1]

My aim in this chapter is to examine the types, especially the illegitimate types, of caring control in health care provision. By 'caring control' I mean medical action and inaction which may frustrate patients' desires or restrict their freedom but which is defended by claiming that it will in the end serve the patients' own best interest. The term 'paternalism' has ordinarily been used in this context, but I shall - for reasons which will become apparent in the course of the paper - forego this usage and employ 'caring control' as my generic term.

The contents of this chapter paper fall roughly into two categories. First, I shall provide an account of the 'anatomy' of caring control: its general definition, an analysis of its types, and an examination of its moral status in different situations. These considerations should make it possible to recognize those instances where medical decisions can be validly justified by appeals to the recipient's own good. Second, I shall review the most important 'pathological' types of caring control – the cases in which references to the patient's own good are used only as a disguise for unjustifiable medical authoritarianism. I shall distinguish three main types of wrongful argument, for which I have coined the terms 'paternalism', 'maternalism' and 'censorism', and discuss their most important features and alleged justifications.

Types of Caring Control

My definition for caring control in medical matters is as follows:

> Caring control takes place when medical professionals or public health authorities refuse to act according to the patient's wishes, or they restrict the patient's freedom or in other ways attempt to influence the patient's behaviour, allegedly in the patient's own best interest.

This is a fairly wide definition in that it covers both practices which can be regarded as strictly authoritarian and policies which would be accepted by the most extreme liberals. Refusals to operate on persons who ask for sterilisation often belong to the former, obviously restrictive, type of control. On the other hand, attempts to influence people's behaviour may include providing them with truthful information, which has not normally been considered as constraining.

The various practices covered by the definition can be classified by examining whether or not they involve coercion, constraint, violations of personal autonomy, or other prima facie immoralities. Two dividing lines – shown in Figure 3.1 – emerge when these criteria are employed.

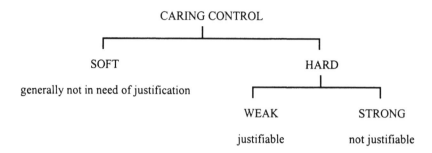

Figure 3.1   The main types of caring control

First, a distinction can be made between those types of control which do in fact include coercive, constraining or harmful elements, and those which do not. I have dubbed these types of caring control 'hard' and 'soft', respectively. Soft interventions such as information campaigns and general education do not normally need separate justifications. Hard caring control, on the other hand, is prima facie condemnable, given that coercion, constraint and the infliction of harm are prima facie condemnable.[2]

A second distinction can be made between two kinds of hard intervention into people's affairs. Some restraints – I have labelled these 'strong' – irrevocably violate the autonomy of persons who are capable of competent decision-making. The initial immorality of these restraints cannot be explained away or justified by appeals to the recipient's own best interest, since it is impossible to further the best interest of competent persons through violations of their autonomy. Autonomy as the self-determination of one's choices and actions is a necessary condition of genuine human happiness, and control which undermines this type of autonomy can never be justified by references to the recipient's own good.

Other interventions, however, despite their coercive or constraining nature, do not in the end amount to actual violations of personal autonomy. These 'weak' instances of caring control can be justified on two conditions. First, they must prevent considerable harm which would otherwise have befallen those whose lives are interfered with. And second, the recipients of the authoritative action in question must be substantially incompetent as regards their ability to make important decisions.

What Justifies Caring Coercion and Constraint?

There are several ways in which persons can be incompetent as regards their ability to make important decisions. Some of the most prominent of these ways are presented in Figure 3.2.

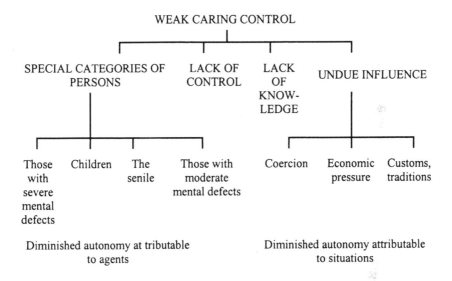

Figure 3.2   Types of justifiable 'hard' caring control[3]

Diminished competence in decision-making is, conceptually, closely related to decreases in the decision-maker's autonomy. Marked reductions in the self-determination of actions and choices are among the most important legitimate grounds for restricting the behaviour of agents in their own best interest. Such reductions of autonomy may be attributable either to the agents themselves or to the situations they find themselves in.

As regards the agents, lack of competence and autonomy in decision-making may originate from at least four factors. People who suffer from severe mental defects may be completely unable to make decisions which could be described as autonomous. Likewise, very young children cannot yet make self-determined choices for themselves, although they are normally expected to develop this ability as they grow up. Senile persons who have irreversibly lost their ability to make autonomous decisions resemble the very young and the mentally defective in that they cannot make decisions concerning their own fates. But assuming that they have in the past been competent agents, their previously expressed wishes should be respected when medical choices are made. Finally, people who have only slight mental defects form a class of their own in that their decision-making capacities may vary considerably over time. In their case, as in the case of normal competent adults, the focus of attention should be fixed on the prevailing circumstances rather than on the personal qualities of the agents involved.

As regards the circumstances, there are at least three factors which may sometimes justify instances of hard caring control.[4] First, one may – due to temporary emotional disturbances – lack sufficient psychological control over one's own choices and actions. This is a situation-related rather than an agent-related matter in that I do not expect sane and rational human beings to be emotionally disturbed unless they have at least some objective grounds for it. On the other hand, of course, different people react very differently to external provocation, so that the decrease of self-determination is also partly attributable to personal factors. Second, lack of knowledge may justify coercive and constraining interventions: individuals cannot make fully autonomous decisions without adequate information concerning the consequences of their actions.[5] Third, even total psychological control combined with complete information does not guarantee self-determined decision-making. Individuals may act under the undue influence of other people, who – intentionally or unintentionally – impose upon them coercive threats, economic pressures or norms dictated by widely accepted customs and traditions. All these elements may undermine the decision-makers' autonomy and self-determination, thereby potentially subjecting them to legitimate coercive control in their own best interest.

Unjustifiable Control: Paternalism, Maternalism and Censorism

It is not necessary for my present purpose to work out a detailed account of the empirical circumstances under which caring control can be justified. It is more important to draw attention to a conceptual point which is often overlooked by defenders of restrictive medical authoritarianism. The point I have in mind is the following. The list of autonomy-diminishing factors presented in Figure 3.2 is meant to specify the rare conditions in which hard caring control, despite its prima facie immorality, can in exceptional cases be justified. Given that coercion and constraint are prima facie condemnable, as liberal theorists assume, the burden of proof rests in each particular case on the person or group who sets out to restrict other people's choices, even if the restrictions were intended to further the recipient's well-being.

Those who defend medical authoritarianism have a different view on the matter. They seem to think that the list of autonomy-diminishing factors provides a general justification for large-scale policies of coercion and constraint in the patients' best interest. According to these defenders of 'strong' control, the burden of proof does not rest on them, but on those health care professionals who leave the choices to the patients. The reasoning behind this view is that in medical situations people are, as a rule, ill, and due to their illness they are incapable of making competent choices concerning treatment. Only a small minority of exceptionally talented decision-makers – most notably physicians themselves – can maintain their competence in the face of disease and injury. The rest of us, so the medical authoritarian claims, must be protected against our own ill-considered choices. Different manifestations of this basic view mark the most important types of strong caring control in medicine and health care.

The three main types of wrongful caring control are presented in Figure 3.3.

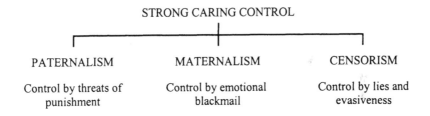

STRONG CARING CONTROL

PATERNALISM	MATERNALISM	CENSORISM
Control by threats of punishment	Control by emotional blackmail	Control by lies and evasiveness

Figure 3.3　Types of strong caring control

The first alternative is that doctors, nurses and public health authorities coerce people, by explicit threats of punishment, into behaviour which can be regarded as rational from the medical viewpoint. This type of control has usually been seen as analogous to the father's control over the family and it has been, subsequently, labelled 'paternalistic'. An example of paternalism would be the state's decision to withdraw certain social benefits, such as public medical services, from those citizens who refuse to assume a healthy life-style as defined by the medical authorities. Paternalism in this limited sense is especially characteristic of the attitudes of public authorities towards the uneducated masses.

The second alternative is that medical professionals resort to emotional blackmail, which is designed to make the patients feel guilty and, eventually, to make them alter their behaviour. Since the term 'paternalism' is widely employed to refer to coercive authoritarianism, I can perhaps coin another family-related metaphor, namely 'maternalism', to refer to this second type of wrongful control. The paternalist is supposed to be the father who threatens to send his children to bed without supper if they behave self-destructively. Following the same logic, the maternalist is the mother who makes it known to her children that she will be extremely sad if they go out and hurt themselves.[6] A medical example of this kind of control would be a nurse who persuades the patients to conform to the hospital rules by an appeal to his or her own hurt feelings. One would expect that maternalism is typically employed in face-to-face situations by relatively low-ranking medical workers who do not have much formal power over their customers.

The third alternative is that health care providers control the behaviour of their clients and patients by telling them half-truths and by giving them evasive answers when they ask sensitive questions. I have labelled this type of caring control 'censorism'. Charges of censorism can most often be directed against practising physicians, although public health authorities are also in a good position to withhold medical information. The paradigmatic case of face-to-face censorism is that of the physician who protects her or his patients by telling them comforting lies. Public health-related censorism, in its turn, is well exemplified by the reluctance with which medical authorities admit that so-called unhealthy products such as alcohol can have beneficial as well as harmful effects.

The Alleged Justifications of Strong Control

The justifications for different types of strong caring control vary considerably. This variety reflects the features and standing of the professional groups which employ authoritarian arguments within medicine and health care. (1) Paternalism is usually defended by appeals to the greater knowledge and experience of the public authorities, who see themselves as acting in loco parentis as regards the rest of society. (2) Arguments for maternalism, in their turn, are founded on the subjective moral convictions of the maternalists themselves and on the claim that emotional persuasion cannot be considered genuinely coercive or constraining. (3) Censorism is a parasitical form of strong control in the sense that it derives its justifications mainly from defences of paternalism and maternalism.

Medical Paternalism

The general strategy employed by public health authorities and others who make it their affair to control people's self-regarding choices is to argue that their constraining actions belong to the category of weak rather than strong caring control. Lack of knowledge is one of the legitimate grounds for restricting people's self-regarding behaviour, and one can claim that the lack of advanced medical knowledge prevailing among the majority of lay persons justifies authoritarian attitudes and regulations. Since, for instance, people do not seem to know about or understand the health risks of the use of alcohol, tobacco and hard drugs, paternalistic interventions which are designed to reduce the consumption of these substances are both legitimate and, from the viewpoint of general welfare, necessary.

The difficulty with this argument is that it proceeds from true premises to false conclusions. It is certainly true that individuals are often less than fully knowledgeable concerning the health hazards of drinking, smoking and drug-taking. But surely the easiest way to rectify the situation would be to pass down the information to the individual citizens, and then let them draw the appropriate conclusions for themselves. These conclusions would not always be the same as the ones made by the medical authorities, but lack of knowledge would nonetheless cease to justify paternalistic regulations. Seen from the liberal viewpoint, public health authorities who prefer prohibitions and restrictions to information campaigns and health education are in fact either mistaken in their views or fundamentally insensitive as regards claims to personal autonomy and individual self-determination. (The various notions and justifications of health education are further examined in chapter 4.)

Faced with counterarguments like this, proponents of medical paternalism usually shift the conversation from the empirical lack of medical knowledge among lay people to the rationality and irrationality of certain choices regarding health and survival. According to some consequentialist theories, agents fail to act rationally if they choose to risk their health or life expectancy in order to achieve immediate pleasures such as those provided by alcohol, tobacco and drugs.[7] Paternalistic intervention, so its proponents argue, is justified because it aims to protect people from the consequences of their own irrational behaviour.

The problem with this view is that irrationality as defined by the consequentialists does not provide sufficient grounds for constraining people's self-regarding behaviour. Agents who are irrational in the specific sense that the consequences of their actions are less than optimal are not necessarily incompetent or nonautonomous. If they are, then interventions are justifiable under the heading of weak caring control. But if the agents do not lack competence or autonomy, then any appeal to their irrationality which is supposed to legitimate paternalism simply begs the question. To call agents irrational in this sense is only another way of saying that the agents are expected to inflict harm on themselves. And what proponents of strong control ought to work out to defend their view in the first instance is a plausible theory to back up the claim that self-destructive behaviour can indeed be legitimately restricted.

One possible link between self-inflicted harm and justifiable constraint is the alleged immorality of harming oneself. There are a number of critical theories as well as common sense views which state that individuals who damage themselves or fail to improve their lot when the opportunity arises are sufficiently unethical to have their actions regulated by law. A theological version of the view states that all human beings belong to God, and that God dislikes the destruction of her or his property. Another, humanistic version of the theory makes an appeal to the needs of our fellow humans: by damaging ourselves we may fail to benefit people whose lives depend on our actions. It has also been argued that we should take our own future selves into account when we make decisions concerning our life-styles, since our future selves are the ones who will suffer the consequences of the choice, not we as we know ourselves at present.[8] Finally, some theorists contend that the moral code which prevails in society is sacrosanct, and it should therefore be enforced by law.[9] All these doctrines are supposedly objective or intersubjective rather than purely subjective in nature. Paternalists normally try to find preexistent intellectual and moral structures to found their views on.

Critical examination quickly reveals the pitfalls of different types of moralistic paternalism. The first view, in addition to having all the deficiencies of theistic theories in general, presents a rather odd picture of the relationship between God and humankind. God, who according to theological accounts should be a loving creator, is depicted as a slaveholder who punishes people for trying to make independent decisions. The second view, in its turn, is problematical in the present context because it cannot be employed to support any kind of caring control. It may, of course, be the case that by harming ourselves we harm other sentient beings, in which case our actions can legitimately be restricted. But the restrictions are in this case justified by harm inflicted on others, not by the harm we may inflict on ourselves.

The third attempt to defend paternalism on ethical grounds, the appeal to our future selves, is interesting, but not convincing enough to make the case for strong control. The problem is that however close the connection between self-inflicted harm and immorality may be, the gap between immorality and the law (or health policy) remains unbridged. There may also be difficulties with the rather peculiar theory of personal identity underlying the view.[10] The fourth defence of paternalism, widely known as the doctrine of legal moralism, has been quite adequately rejected in the literature.[11] Under closer scrutiny the doctrine is either reduced to the principle of other-regarding harm or to the principle of offence.[12] In the former case, caring control remains unsupported by the doctrine. In the latter case, an auxiliary theory would be needed to show that pure moral offensiveness can justify legal regulations. Up to the present, however, no successful efforts have been made to formulate such a theory.[13] On the whole, it seems that paternalism as a specific form of strong caring control cannot be legitimated by moral or moralistic considerations.

Medical Maternalism

The defenders of the second form of strong caring control, maternalism, often build their cases on the alleged fact that emotional persuasion can never be coercive or constraining. If this view is correct, maternalism is not a form of hard caring control in the first place, and no separate justification is required for it.

Unfortunately for the maternalists, however, the correctness of the view can be challenged. The theory of freedom and constraint underlying maternalistic reasoning states that only physical hindrances and coercion by threats of physical violence can restrict human liberty. Emotional persuasion, according to the view, does not curtail liberty since the recipient can always refuse to yield to the wishes of the persuader. But this account of freedom and constraint is clearly untenable. Assuming that psychological pressures cannot in fact restrict individual freedom because they can be refused, the same argument can be applied to physical hindrances and coercion as well. Prisoners must, admittedly, adjust their spatial movements and daily routines to the prison walls and prison rules, but they can refuse to repent their deeds. And those coerced by threats of physical violence are always free to choose the physical violence instead of submitting to the coercer's wishes. Surely it should not be inferred from these observations that force and coercion have no influence on human liberty.

An alternative theory of freedom and constraint gives a more balanced view of the relationship between coercion, force, and restrictions of liberty. According to this theory, individuals are free when – and to the degree that – their options, or action alternatives, are unrestricted.[14] People who are imprisoned have only few of their pre-conviction options open to them, and they can therefore be regarded as substantially unfree. Those who are faced with threats of physical violence are free in the sense that the combined choice which consists of (i) rejecting the demands of the threatener and (ii) suffering the consequences is open to them even after the threat. On the other hand, they are not free to select the combined option which was available to them before the threat and which consisted of (i) ignoring the threatener's wishes but (ii) remaining unharmed. Drawing an analogy to this latter case, maternalistic actions can be seen as threats of psychological harm. The recipients of maternalistic intervention are free to reject the directives given to them, but the rejection makes them unfree to live without the awareness of the pain they may have inflicted on another person.

Consider the case of the nurse who persuades his patients to conform to the hospital rules by referring to his own hurt feelings. The procedure may involve verbal communication, i.e. the nurse can say, 'Look here, Mrs Doe, if you don't stop parachuting from the hospital roof in the small hours, your arm will never get better and I shall be very sad.' More often the message is conveyed by nonverbal means such as sighs and depressed gestures. Whatever the channel of communication, however, the first effect of maternalistic action is the same on almost every recipient. The patient becomes aware of the fact that by doing what she wants to do she will hurt other people's feelings. The implications of this awareness may, of course, vary considerably depending on the patient's mental constitution and moral views. But the initial awareness concerning the situation is unavoidable, and the seeds of guilt are thus always sown. As for the constraint caused by the intervention, the recipient is unfree to return to the state of pleasant ignorance which was unconditionally available to her before she was subjected to maternalistic action.

The maternalist can respond to these considerations by focusing on the actual effects of emotional persuasion on different kinds of people. According to the defence, there are two alternative reactions to maternalistic control, neither of which supports its rejection. First, there are individuals who remain practically untouched by the intervention, since it evokes no guilty feelings in them. In their case, restrictions of individual liberty do not occur, and justifications are not needed. Second, there are also individuals in whom emotional persuasion does evoke guilt. But this guilt is a product of the recipient's own awareness concerning the immorality of her or his actions. No options are restricted unless the recipients themselves feel that what they do is wrong. And it can surely be argued that choices which are seen as unethical even by those who make them need not be fully respected.

Despite the initial plausibility of this argument, there are serious flaws in it. The fact that some individuals remain untouched by emotional appeals does not necessarily mean that their behaviour is immune to blame. It is equally possible that what they do is wrong and they know it, but they do not care about it. Even if maternalism were justified, it would in these cases be ineffective. On the other hand, the fact that other individuals do feel guilt does not prove that their actions are genuinely immoral. Sensitive persons often react strongly to other people's emotional distress, and they may nurture guilty feelings simply because they cannot meet the demands of others, however unreasonable these demands may be. In these cases maternalistic interventions are self-fulfilling in the sense that the maternalists themselves create the subjective moral universe within which the recipient's guilt occurs.

The maternalist's last defence is to argue that those controlled by persuasion would otherwise cause inconvenience by their unruly behaviour. In the hospital example three interpretations can be given to this argument, but none of them makes the case for maternalism as a form of strong caring control. First, the nurse could claim that the patient herself will in the long run be inconvenienced if she does not comply with the hospital rules. If this claim is intended to refer to the guilt evoked in the patient, the harm is produced by the nurse himself, and cannot be employed to support strong control without provoking charges of circularity. If, again, the point is that the patient's recovery may be delayed by disobedience, the choice is obviously the patient's to make. Second, it can be argued that disturbances and delays adversely affect the daily routines of the ward, thereby jeopardizing the well-being of other patients. In those cases where this is true, restrictions may indeed be appropriate. But what justifies them is harm inflicted on other persons, not the patient's own best interest. Third, the most probable interpretation to the argument is that the nurse himself will be inconvenienced by the patient's behaviour. If this is the case, there may occasionally be some weak other-regarding grounds for controlling the patient's actions. But it is also possible that the demands made by the nurse only reflect his own egoism. After all, a nurse who cannot bear to be inconvenienced by her or his patients stands professionally on rather shaky grounds.

Medical Censorism

The third form of strong caring control, medical censorism, typically assumes the form of linguistic elusiveness and evasiveness. Especially physicians tend to hide the meaning of their sentences behind technical expressions and Latinate terms. In addition, physicians as well as other medical professionals and health authorities employ silence and verbal patronizing as methods of preventing or evading questions they do not wish to answer.

The excessive use of medical Latin in the doctor-patient relationship is often simply due to the physician's professional incompetence. In the case of young medical practitioners such elusiveness may be symptomatic of a lack of medical knowledge and experience. This form of censorism is, at least theoretically, curable by time. But even experienced medical professionals may sometimes be unable to communicate their opinions to patients in plain English. Their problem, which culminates in their inadvertent censorism, may be that they lack the socio-linguistic skills which ought to be required of truly competent health-care providers. In these cases it is easy to see how censorism as a pathological form of caring control emerges from insufficient medical or linguistic skills.

But there are also physicians who, despite their competence to communicate with their patients, deliberately choose to be elusive and evasive. Latinate language is one of the methods they can employ when they want to give uninformative answers to sensitive questions. Other types of evasion include lies, half-truths, baby talk and silence. Some theorists would like to exclude silence from the list on the ground that unasked questions need not be answered: as long as physicians adequately respond to those questions that the patient actually poses, they can ignore the potential questions that the patient might, given the opportunity, wish to ask. The argument in favour of this view is to claim that acts and omissions are morally asymmetrical in the sense that while harmful acts are morally condemnable, harmful omissions are not. But the theoretical standing of this view is unclear, and the distinction cannot hold the weight of the argument. If the consequences of not informing the patient about his medical condition are exactly as undesirable as the consequences of lying to him, there seems to be little reason to distinguish morally between the two cases. If, again, it could be proved that lying usually brings about more harm than silence does, this would only prove that most acts of lying are more condemnable than most omissions to inform the patient. It would not prove that silence in the face of the patient's unasked questions could be excluded from the list of methods of wrongful medical authoritarianism.

The proponents of censorism often defend their views by appeals to the arguments introduced in the context of maternalism and paternalism. First, since censorism is a purely verbal form of caring control, it can be argued that it does not involve coercion, constraint or violations of autonomy and it should therefore be regarded as a form of soft control. Second, even if prima facie violations of autonomy do occur occasionally, these can be justified by the fact that the recipients are less than fully autonomous in the first place.

Withholding information from patients who could not use it adequately in any case belongs to the category of justifiable, weak caring control.

The arguments from lack of constraint and diminished autonomy are, however, as erroneous here as they are when employed to defend maternalism and paternalism. As for the point that censorism is a form of soft control, it should be obvious to anybody that lies and half-truths prevent the recipients from informed decision-making, thereby grossly violating their autonomy.[15] Although censorism does not involve the use of coercion or physical force, it is hardly plausible to claim that it does not constrain the recipients' choices and actions. The situation is slightly different when it comes to the allegation that lying and witholding medical information can be justified by appeals to the recipients' lack of competence or autonomy. Some patients are indeed incapable of considered decision-making no matter how well the physician informs them about their condition. But the fact remains that when this is the case, medical authorities are entitled to practice weak, not strong caring control. Given that individuals can be said to have a prima facie right to self-determination in matters which concern solely or mainly themselves, caring control can be justifiable in exceptional situations, but it must not become a routine solution in medicine and health care.

Another argument for censorism in health care is based on the fact that medical knowledge is limited. This argument has two forms, depending on the level of ignorance assumed. One can either presume that medical knowledge is sometimes limited or that it is always limited. The former claim is in itself noncontroversial, but it does not entail the normative results that censorists would like it to entail. The latter claim, in its turn, is both controversial by itself and difficult to utilize in the censorist's argumentation.

In the first formulation it is assumed that medical knowledge is sometimes limited. Whatever the physician's intentions about informing the patient, there are cases in which medical professionals simply cannot tell for certain how the patient's condition is going to develop. How should physicians act in such circumstances? Proponents of censorism hold that patients always expect the physician to tell them something which is convincing and seems knowledgeable. If this were true, then doctors would appear to have an obligation to resort to lies and half-truths whenever their knowledge is incomplete. But it is by no means obvious that patients always expect to hear convincing and comforting lies. There may have been a time when people did not wish to know about their exact predicament, and preferred cosy lies to the unpleasantness of truth. But nowadays a growing number of people seem to have revised their thinking. They want to know where the limits of factual knowledge are drawn and where values, hopes and fears can legitimately enter their decision-making.

In the second formulation it is assumed that medical knowledge is always limited, and to such a degree that there are, in fact, no absolute truths to be told to the patients. According to the proponents of censorism, this implies that the only criterion the physician ought to respect in her work is the influence her actions – including her verbal communications – have on the patient. If, for instance, lies improve the patient's condition, then they are legitimate. This view can, however, be challenged on two accounts. First, although there may be no absolute truths in life, physicians do know a great deal about the development of diseases and the effectiveness of various treatments. It does not correspond with facts to presume that medical professionals are totally ignorant. Second, even if physicians were ignorant, it would not follow that censorism is acceptable. On the contrary, if medical professionals do not possess the expert knowledge that they have for decades claimed to possess, their fraudulence should be exposed to the general public. Individuals are entitled to know that they have been treated by quacks, if that is the case.

Conclusions

It seems, then, that all three forms of 'strong' caring control are unacceptable in modern societies. Public health authorities cannot plausibly argue that lack of knowledge would justify large-scale policies of medical paternalism. Nurses and other lower-level health care workers cannot truthfully claim that their maternalistic interventions should be regarded as mere offers of friendly advice. Physicians cannot possibly show that their own lack of knowledge entails a justification for censorism. And similar considerations are valid as regards paternalistic nurses and doctors, maternalistic authorities and physicians, and censoristic nurses and public officials.

When liberal theorists criticize medical authoritarianism, they have primarily focused their attention on paternalism. The probable reason for this limited viewpoint is that explicit coercion is more visible than emotional persuasion and evasiveness in parting with information. However, once the three forms of wrongful caring control have been distinguished, it becomes immediately clear that paternalism in the strict sense is only the tip of the iceberg. It is, no doubt, unethical to coerce or force treatments or life-styles upon patients whose decisions to refuse these treatments or life-styles are essentially autonomous. But it may be even more unethical to exploit the finer feelings of the patients to achieve some dubious institutional ends, or to withhold important medical information from them. When patients are faced with straightforward threats of violence, they can at least recognize the injustice and protest against the treatment, but it is considerably more difficult to defend oneself against institutionalized lies and half-truths. More attention, therefore, should be given to the neglected forms of wrongful medical authoritarianism that I have labelled maternalism and censorism.

Notes

An early version of this chapter was presented in *The Participant Patient: Patient or Agent in Health Care Decision Making?*, the annual conference of the Society for Applied Philosophy, 24-26 May 1991, Isle-of-Thorns, Sussex. I am grateful to all those participants of the meeting who offered useful ideas during the discussion period. My thanks are also due to Dr Mark Shackleton, Lecturer in English, University of Helsinki, for checking my English.

1   The principles prevailing in medical ethics are well described in T.L. Beauchamp and J.F. Childress, *Principles of Biomedical Ethics* (second edition, New York: Oxford University Press, 1983). On the problems of beneficent control against the wishes of the controlled, see, e.g., J.F. Childress, *Who Should Decide? Paternalism in Health Care* (New York and Oxford: Oxford University Press, 1982); J. Kleinig, *Paternalism* (Manchester: Manchester University Press, 1983); H. Häyry, *The Limits of Medical Paternalism* (London and New York: Routledge, 1991).

2   It is not a matter for this paper to show that coercion, constraint and violations of autonomy are prima facie condemnable. For a defence of the view, see, e.g., Häyry 1991, pp. 44-50.

3   The division presented in the figure originates from C.L. Ten, 'Paternalism and morality', *Ratio* 13 (1971): 56-66, pp. 61-63.

4   I use the cautious form 'may sometimes justify' advisedly: the fact that there are justifiable instances of hard caring control (i.e. justified paternalism in the wide sense) is quite compatible with the view that large-scale *policies* of caring control are always illegitimate.

5   This is presumably the message of J.S. Mill's oft-quoted bridge example, where Mill allows us to prevent a person from crossing a bridge, provided that the person does not know (as we do) that the bridge is dangerous - J.S. Mill, *On Liberty* (1859), in R. Wollheim (ed.), *Three Essays* (Oxford: Oxford University Press, 1975), p. 118.

6   Notice that the inherent sexism of this metaphor is only a counterpart to the sexism of the paternalism metaphor which has been widely employed by

feminist authors who have regarded wrongful authoritativeness as an exclusively male quality. As I see it, however, members of all sexes and genders are equally capable of patronizing (or 'matronizing') their fellow human beings, and it is therefore only fair that mothers as well as fathers get their fair share of the terminology of perverted 'caring control'.

7   See, e.g., D. Parfit, *Reasons and Persons* (Oxford and New York: Oxford University Press, 1986), pp. 317–321. My thanks are due to Dr Roger Crisp (St Anne's College, Oxford) for drawing my attention to this point.

8   Parfit 1986, pp. 317–321.

9   The classical statement of this view is P. Devlin, *The Enforcement of Morals* (Oxford and New York: Oxford University Press, 1965), ch. 1.

10   For an account of the 'reductionist' view of personal identity, see Parfit 1986, p. 321. For a critique of the view in the context of strong caring control, see Häyry 1991, pp. 131–137.

11   For critiques of Devlin's view, see, e.g., R. Wollheim, 'Crime, sin, and Mr. Justice Devlin', *Encounter* **13** (1959): 34–40; H.L.A. Hart, *Law, Liberty and Morality* (Oxford and New York: Oxford University Press, 1963); R. Dworkin, *Taking Rights Seriously* (London: Duckworth, 1977), ch. 10.

12   See, e.g., Häyry 1991, pp. 102–104.

13   A possible counterexample is J. Feinberg's *Offence to Others* (New York and Oxford: Oxford University Press, 1985), which defends the view that offences as well as harms are wrongs which can be regulated by criminal law. But Feinberg's point is related to offences which cause actual unpleasant inconvenience, not to 'pure' moral offences (see, e.g., p. 49). Feinberg's view can only be employed to support the view that genuine offence to others sometimes comes so close to harm that it should be checked by legislation. His arguments do not support moralistic paternalism.

14   This theory in its modern form was formulated in S.I. Benn and W.L. Weinstein, 'Being free to act, and being a free man', *Mind* **80** (1971): 194–211.

15   'Autonomy' should be understood here as the individual's capacity and right to make self-determined choices regarding personally important matters.

4 Health Education, the Ideal Observer and Personal Autonomy

Health education is often seen simply as a means of promoting the physical wellbeing of the community. Within this model health is regarded as a condition which is worth pursuing, and education is thought of as an instrument which helps to bring about that good condition. The idea sounds, to a certain degree, plausible. But what advocates of this view have generally failed to note is that the only proper justification for the model can be found in utility calculations which do not respect the autonomy of individuals. If health education is seen by public authorities as a mechanism by which people's health can be improved without their considered and explicit consent, the authorities can be led to act immorally, and in some cases also irrationally.

My aim in this chapter is to clarify and to justify these points, and to sketch an ethically more acceptable way of looking at health education. I shall begin by formulating a tentative argument for the mechanistic view of health education, and by defending this argument against some of the criticisms that can be levelled at it. I shall then, however, go on to refute the direct appeal to mechanical health promotion by reference to its ill effects on personal self-determination. This leads up to an analysis of the content and value of autonomy in different philosophical approaches, and I shall conclude by outlining my own definition of morally desirable health education.

The Argument for the Mechanical Promotion of Health

If health education is seen directly as a means to promote people's physical wellbeing, the most coherent argument in its favour is probably the following:

(P1)   Human practices are right if and only if they aim at producing the maximum amount of good, or, the maximum number of good states of affairs.

57

(P2)   States of affairs are good if and only if they are regarded as good by a calm, well-informed, rational individual – an 'ideal observer'.

(P3)   In health-related matters, public health authorities can be seen as the closest equivalent to the ideal observer.

(P4)   The health of the population is regarded as good by the public health authorities.

(P5)   The public authorities believe that health education promotes the health of the population.

(CL)   Therefore, it is right to provide people with health education.

Due to the qualifications in premises three and five – the references to 'close equivalence' and the 'beliefs of the authorities' – the conclusion could be formulated in less stringent terms. But given that the rightness of human actions is based on the best estimates we can come by at the time of the choice, not on absolute certainty, the premises also support the more rigid conclusion.[1]

Does Health Education Promote Health?

The validity of the belief mentioned in the fifth premise (P5) can be challenged by arguing that health education falls into two categories, neither of which can actually be expected to promote health. The first type consists of the dissemination of information without attempts to appeal to people's emotions and anxieties. This kind of education can be ignored all too easily, and the only people who notice the warnings issued by the authorities and take them seriously are those who are already concerned about their health, and who would have acted in accordance with the advice even without the official efforts. Their wellbeing will not be significantly promoted by extensive health education, and neither will the wellbeing of others.

The second type, the objection continues, aims at behaviour changes through people's fears and concerns, preferably without the critical intervention of their intellectual faculties. Education like this is directed at convincing individuals that they are sinning against the great values of health and physical fitness if they practice such vices as smoking, drinking, eating rich food and foregoing physical exercise. The only result that public authorities can achieve by taking this route is that they increase and heighten feelings of guilt and inadequacy among the population. Some people will change their behaviour patterns, but the small gain received in terms of physical health will be counteracted by the huge losses incurred in the form of mental anguish and the enforcement of moralistic attitudes.

This objection contains some truth, but it does not refute the mechanistic model of health education. Public authorities can argue that although pure information does not necessarily change attitudes, it does bring benefits to the wise who already try to take care of their own wellbeing. For instance, the knowledge concerning the ways in which the acquired immune deficiency syndrome, AIDS, can be contracted reportedly changed sexual behaviour among gay men in San Francisco by 1985, that is, quite early on in the history of the pandemic.[2] It can also be argued, although the public authorities usually avoid doing so, that the general improvement in the health status of the population fully compensates for any minor inconveniences that are linked with the production of guilty feelings. The additional life years that can be secured by scaring individuals into healthier life-styles are far more important than the temporary and irrational depressions that some people choose to nurture when they are confronted with the truth.

Liberty or Health?

It can be plausibly maintained, then, that health education does promote the physical wellbeing of the population, and that the fifth premise of the argument is valid. But the opponents of the mechanistic model can also argue that the fourth premise (4) is questionable, since many other states of affairs besides health can be regarded as good in a calm and dispassionate analysis. Public health authorities should, qua public authorities, recognize that at least civil liberty is among the values which ought to be protected by policy makers. A firm commitment to liberty, so the opponents can argue, should imply that the freedom of individuals to smoke, drink, eat fatty foods and avoid exercise annuls the official obligations and entitlements to interfere with the self-chosen life-styles of the adult population.

The strength of this objection depends on the definition of freedom it is based upon.[3] If freedom is equated simply with the absence of external constraints to do or to have something the individual wishes to do or to have, the criticism rests on rather shaky grounds. Two questions arise here. First, what is it that people are supposed to want and public authorities are supposed to hinder them from having? The only things that can be achieved by unhealthy life-styles are a few transitory pleasures now, and an increased probability of illness and premature death in the future. Can this be what people genuinely want? From the viewpoint of the ideal observer, the authorities are surely correct when they try to prevent people from harming themselves so unwisely.

The second question concerns the extent to which the authorities can be expected to succeed in their attempts. From what should people be free to drink, smoke, glut themselves and be idle? Health education does not prevent people from doing these things – it merely informs them about the risks that can be attached to them. Even in societies where health education is widely practised, individuals are to all intents and purposes free from external constraints to choose their own ways of living. The only force that can make them change their habits is, in the end, their own deteriorating health. Although people's civil liberties must be protected, health authorities can remark, there is no point in protecting them at the expense of people's future freedom to make choices concerning their lives.

The Ideal Observer vs. Personal Autonomy

The appeal to liberty does not refute the argument for mechanical health promotion as long as the first three premises of the argument (1–3) remain unchallenged. If it is our duty to maximize the good *and* if what is good must be defined by the ideal observer *and* if the public authorities are the closest anybody can get to the ideal observer, then it is, regardless of our own opinions, our duty as citizens to follow the guidelines set by the officials through health education, and it is their obligation to see to it that we do.

The paternalistic suppositions of this norm can, however, be questioned. A human practice is not necessarily right just because it happens to maximize the good as seen by the public authorities, however calm, well-informed and rational they may be. It is, namely, possible to argue that individuals are entitled, by right, to make their own decisions, when these decisions concern only or primarily themselves.[4] If this is sound, then people can have a moral duty to maximize the wellbeing – or at least minimize the suffering – of others, while they can quite legitimately make choices which are bad for their own health. The greater knowledge and impartiality of the authorities guarantees their expertise in the epistemic sense, but when it comes to matters which fall within the scope of people's personal self-determination and autonomy, they are morally on their own.

What is Autonomy?

The notion of autonomy has two main interpretations, which are related to what Isaiah Berlin called the positive and negative concepts of liberty.[5] Those who uphold the *positive* concept of liberty believe that freedom means the presence of certain rationally, emotionally, politically or morally correct restrictions. Their idea of personal autonomy is that individuals can achieve genuine self-determination only by subjecting their lusts and desires to the universal human will to be moral, or to their own vital need to live in an organized society. The former, moral solution was advocated by Immanuel Kant,[6] and the latter, more political model can be found in the works of Jean-Jacques Rousseau.[7]

The defenders of the *negative* concept of liberty usually argue that freedom means simply the absence of restrictions. If this view is taken to refer only to positive, external restrictions,[8] then the content of personal autonomy is either reduced to freedom from coercion, which is the libertarian answer,[9] or it is borrowed from the Kantian doctrine, which was John Rawls' solution.[10]

But if the restrictions in question are also extended to negative and internal constraints like lack of self-control, then autonomy can be seen in a different light. Joel Feinberg, for instance, has given four meanings to 'autonomy' when the term is applied to individuals. These are (i) 'the *capacity* [or potential ability] to govern oneself'; (ii) 'the *actual condition* of self-government and its associated virtues'; (iii) 'an *ideal of character* derived from that conception'; and (iv) 'the *right* of self-determination'.[11] In this model autonomy can be seen, then, depending on the context, either as a potential, an actuality, a value, or a norm.

The Value of Autonomy: False Starts

The value of autonomy within the views which rely on the positive concept of liberty is based on the idea that what is rational is always preferable to what is not. In Rousseau's model the idea is that the value of autonomy, or freedom to live in an ideal society while obeying its rational rules, is contingent on the value of the ideal society itself. Human beings living in a society can only be truly happy when everybody has submitted 'his person and his power under the supreme direction of the general will',[12] and autonomy is, therefore, valuable only when it involves an absolute submission to the rules set by the authorities. Kant's point, in its turn, is that the value of autonomy is linked with the ultimate value of rational morality.

Instead of submitting one's decisions to the socially determined general will, the Kantian individual is bound to obey the transcendental 'real' will, which must control people's own 'empirical' wills.

In Rousseau's theory the value of an individual's autonomy is undermined by its social determination. In the framework of health education, his view could be employed to *defend* the mechanical promotion of physical wellbeing more naturally than to criticize it. If society requires health of its members, then people should not make unhealthy choices against the advice given by the authorities.

Kant's doctrine, again, can be interpreted in two ways, neither of which is helpful here. The first reading follows Rousseau, and states that individuals ought to be forced into making rational choices, whatever ideas they themselves may have. The second contends that since autonomy must be found within the person, it is not possible to coerce people into making genuinely self-determined decisions. Within the first reading, the choices made by actual individuals count for next to nothing in health care policy-making, within the second the authorities have no way of influencing the autonomous decisions of moral persons.

In liberal theories, which place their trust in the negative concept of liberty, autonomy can be valuable either as a means to something else or as an end in itself.[13] A prominent option is to claim that the self-determination of one's actions, choices and life-plans is essential to the pursuit of well-being and happiness. John Stuart Mill, for instance, argued in the wider context of general policy that 'a state which dwarfs its men, in order that they may be more docile instruments in its hands even for beneficial purposes, will find that with small men no great things can really be accomplished'.[14] Mill's point seems to be that the promotion of liberty and autonomy is a causal factor without which it would be impossible to bring about genius and industriousness, which in their turn are necessary prerequisites of material welfare and cultural greatness.

The problem with this approach in health education is that the causal connections it presumes defy any real proof. It can be claimed that people are, in the end, healthier if they are allowed to make their own choices concerning their life-styles. But it can equally well be argued that the health of the population is best secured by paternalistic interventions and benevolent manipulation. The instrumental value of personal self-determination remains, inevitably, obscure.[15]

The Intrinsic Value of Autonomy

When it comes to defending the *intrinsic* value of autonomy, some philosophers have thought that it is helpful to think about the imaginary social order described by Aldous Huxley in his satirical novel *Brave New World*.[16] Huxley's New World is a peaceful, stable and health-oriented society from which all standard sources of conflict have been removed by eliminating family ties and other close human bonds, natural reproduction, restrictions of sexual freedom, pain, anguish, suffering, illness, old age and the experience of death. Instead, human embryos and fetuses develop in a hatchery during their prenatal period, after which they are hypnopaedically programmed to the tasks, opinions and values of their caste. Adult inhabitants of the New World lead a happy life in the sense that they are content, and there are always pleasures available to them when they want or need them. The main forms of recreation are sensual entertainment, games, promiscuous sex and the use of psychoactive drugs. Since the society has rather conclusively determined every decision an inhabitant is apt to make, the very idea of autonomy, however, is alien to the new order.

Most people would presumably not think that the society described by Huxley would be an ideal place to live in. One of the main reasons for this is that the happiness enjoyed in the Brave New World does not seem to be the kind of happiness that makes human life worth living. Pleasures, admittedly, could be experienced by individuals, but not in a considered manner, not in a manner that would enable the individual to be proud of a good choice, thereby multiplying the value of the experience. It seems that contentment without autonomy would be less valuable than happiness accompanied by self-government, and this connection can be seen to give autonomy its intrinsic worth.

How can Autonomy be Respected in Health Education?

Granted that autonomy is intrinsically valuable and that it should be respected in health policies as well as in other areas of life, what does this mean for health education? Gerald Dworkin has presented a workable list of attitudes, norms and preferences which are usually associated with respect for autonomy in all policy-making. These are:

(1) We have favourable attitudes towards those methods of influence which support the self-respect and dignity of those who are being influenced.
    [...]

(2) Methods of influence which are destructive of the ability to individuals to reflect rationally on their interests should not be used. [...]

(3) Methods should not be used which affect in fundamental ways the personal identity of individuals. [...]

(4) Methods which rely essentially on deception, on keeping the agent in ignorance of relevant facts, are to be avoided. [...]

(5) Modes of influence which are not physically intrusive are preferable to those which are. [...]

(6) There will be some restrictions on the time in which the changes take place and the ability of the agent to resist the effects of various modes of influence. [...]

(7) We prefer methods of influence which work through the cognitive and affective structure of the agent, which require the active participation of the agent in producing the change, to those which short-circuit the desires and beliefs of the agent and make him a passive recipient of the changes.[17]

Although Dworkin's points are rather general, many of them can be employed almost directly to the assessment and redefinition of health education.

The following practical guidelines, which are partly overlapping, are perhaps the most important that can be derived from Dworkin's ideas:

(a) Modes of health education that violate the autonomy of individuals should not be encouraged.

(b) Self-evidently, health education should never involve corporal punishment.

(c) Modes of health education that enhance the autonomy of individuals ought to be encouraged.

(d) Health education should not be frightening or overly emotional, nor should it evoke feelings of guilt or build up undue pressures in the life-styles chosen by individuals.

(e) Health education should ideally disseminate truthful information about the causes of ill health and the dangers confronting people at home, at the work place and elsewhere.

(f) Since lying and deception are to be condemned, public health authorities should not conceal, or omit to inform people about, the good effects of life-styles which are regarded as unhealthy, for instance, the advantages of consuming moderate quantities of alcohol.

In one form or another, all Dworkin's points are at least partially covered with these principles.

If all these norms are taken seriously, health education ceases to be a mechanical means to promote people's physical wellbeing, and becomes an autonomy-enhancing method of health policy. The best way to define this policy is to say that, instead of trying to make people healthy against their own wishes, health education should aim at making people aware of the *conditions* of their own health. Individuals cannot be legitimately forced into physical wellbeing regardless of their self-determined decisions, but they can, and should, be informed about the factors that are relevant to their life-styles and health. The availability of information can eventually lead to the improvement of the physical wellbeing of the population, but if it does, this should be treated as a bonus, not as the primary goal of health education.

Notes

An earlier version of this chapter was presented at the *10th Annual Conference of the European Society for Philosophy of Medicine and Health Care*, Vienna, 14–17 August, 1996. My thanks are due to Dr Mark Shackleton, Lecturer in English, University of Helsinki, for checking my English.

1   The ethical theory on which the argument is based can be labelled as 'classical' or 'modern' utilitarianism in the sense defined in M. Häyry, *Liberal Utilitarianism and Applied Ethics* (London and New York: Routledge, 1994).

2   L. McKusick, W. Horstman and T.J. Coates, 'AIDS and sexual behavior reported by gay men in San Francisco', *American Journal of Public Health* 75 (1985): 493–496.

3   On different definitions of 'freedom', see, e.g., H. Häyry, *The Limits of Medical Paternalism* (London and New York: Routledge, 1991), pp. 26–31.

4   The classical statement of this view can be found in John Stuart Mill's *On Liberty* (1859), in R. Wollheim (ed.), *Three Essays* (Oxford: Oxford University Press, 1975), pp. 14–15.

5   I. Berlin, 'Two concepts of liberty' (1958), reprinted in his *Four Essays on Liberty* (Oxford: Oxford University Press, 1969).

6   I. Kant, *Grundlegung zur Metaphysik der Sitten* (1786) ed. by M. Thom (Leipzig: Reclam, 1983); I. Kant, *Kritik der praktischen Vernunft* (1788), ed. by M. Thom (Leipzig: Reclam, 1983).

7   J.-J. Rousseau, *The Social Contract or Principles of Political Right* (1762), in *The Social Contract and Discourses*, transl. G.D.H. Cole, ed. by J.H. Brumfitt and J.C. Hall (London: J.M. Dent & Sons Ltd., 1986).

8   In Joel Feinberg's terminology, positive constraints work by being present and negative constraints by being absent. The former include 'headaches, obsessive thoughts, and compulsive desires' as well as barred windows, locked doors and pointed bayonets'; the latter class consists of things such as 'ignorance, weakness, and deficiencies in talent or skill along with 'lack of money, lack of transportation, and lack of weapons'. External constraints come from outside a person's mind-body continuum, internal constraints are a part of it. See J. Feinberg, *Social Philosophy* (Englewood Cliffs, New Jersey: Prentice-Hall, 1973), p. 13.

9   Robert Nozick's libertarian classic *Anarchy, State and Utopia* (Oxford and New York: Basil Blackwell, 1974), for instance, does not even list the term 'autonomy' in its index.

10   J. Rawls, *A Theory of Justice* (Oxford: Oxford University Press, 1972), pp. 252 ff.

11   J. Feinberg, *Harm to Self* (New York and Oxford: Oxford University Press, 1986), p. 28. Italics in (i), (ii) and (iii) original, in (iv) added.

12   Rousseau 1986, p. 192 (italics deleted).

13   The value of autonomy can also be nonexistent like in libertarianism, where the concept has no independent meaning.

14   Mill 1975, p. 141.

15   As regards the link between autonomy and genius, for instance, Berlin (1969, p. 128) has noted that severely disciplined communities such as the Calvinists of New England have given birth to at least as many geniuses as more tolerant ones. And the material welfare of restrictive societies has not always been lesser than the welfare of liberal communities.

16   A. Huxley, *Brave New World* (1932), ed. by M.S. Ellis (Harlow, Essex: Longman, 1983).

17   G. Dworkin, 'Moral autonomy', in H.T. Engelhardt, Jr. and D. Callahan (eds.), *Morals, Science and Sociality Vol. III: The Foundations of Ethics and Its Relationship to Science* (New York: The Hastings Center, 1978), pp. 164-166.

5 Preventive Medicine and the Welfare of the Population

In addition to face-to-face clinical paternalism and public health education, the populations of industrialized societies are also subject to more delicate and far more extensive forms of possibly paternalistic intervention. These include, most notably, laws regulating dangerous behaviour in everyday life, regulations concerning the manufacture, advertising, sale and consumption of drugs and intoxicating substances, and preventive medical and socio-political measures such as quarantines, vaccinations and plumbing. In fact, a surprisingly large part of these regulations and activities are ethically unproblematical, either because there are good non-paternalistic grounds for upholding and approving them, or because their paternalism is, measured by the standards of freedom and autonomy, clearly legitimate or clearly illegitimate, as the case may be.

Seat Belt and Crash Helmet Laws

As regards laws regulating *dangerous everyday behaviour*, there are two examples which have often dominated philosophical discussions on the topic, namely driving a car without using a seat belt and riding a motorcycle without wearing a crash helmet. The liberal assessment of sanctioning these practices is simple: unless the motorists can be expected to inflict harm on other people by their behaviour, there are no legitimate grounds for constraint. Minors excluded, individuals are entitled to apparently stupid, reckless and irresponsible choices, such as the rejection of simple safety precautions in traffic, if the risk taken is mainly or entirely self-regarding.

Three kinds of argument can be put forward, however, to prove that the seemingly self-regarding nature of unsafe motoring is an illusion, and that other people are, after all, harmed as a result of fatal accidents.[1] First, according to what can be called 'the threshold argument', people driving without seat belts and safety helmets present a threat against society as a whole, since in fatal accidents the social fabric will be deprived of able-bodied citizens, whose future contribution will be lost, and who will possibly create an unnecessary burden for the health care system. Second, there is the argument from indirect harm, stating that families and friends will be disturbed and economically inconvenienced by a refusal to take all the necessary precautions. And third, it can also be suggested that harm will be inflicted on other motorists, who have to see the crushed skulls and twisted bodies, and on the people who are responsible for washing away the blood and cleaning up the debris.

But these attempts to justify restrictions are inadequate. The main difficulty, and one which the three attempts have in common, is that almost all serious traffic accidents have the effects listed here, quite regardless of the use of helmets, and often regardless of the use of seat belts as well. In fact, it could well be claimed against the first two arguments that the helmet is a particularly controversial device, as it covers the skull but leaves the spine unprotected. The 'unnecessary health care costs' increase considerably if the patient survives with serious spinal damage instead of bashing her head in and passing quietly away, and the 'psychological burden on the family and friends' will also be prolonged. It may, of course, be that the patients themselves would prefer being alive even if it meant permanent paralysis, but such a preference would be self-regarding rather than other-regarding, and therefore could not be utilized in non-paternalistic argumentation.

Quarantines

Moving on to regulations and practices which are more conspicuously medical in nature, *quarantines* – as traditional and recognized instruments of preventing disease – draw their justification from the public good instead of the good of the ones whose freedom is restricted or autonomy violated. It was definitely not for the sailors' sake that the ships arriving in port and suspected of carrying contagious diseases were held in isolation from the shore for a period of forty days, nor was it for their own best interest that AIDS patients in Sweden were until recently transported into an isolated nursing home on an island. Quarantines and quarantine-like measures such as home arrest, electronic surveillance, compulsory hospitalization and imprisonment are justifiable, *if* they are justifiable, by an appeal to the potential harm inflicted on other people by carriers of communicable diseases.[2]

There are, of course, many qualifications which reduce the ethical acceptability of isolation policies in real-life situations: the threat posed on others may be symbolic rather than concrete (as is often the case with 'mental illness');[3] the isolation can amount to the life imprisonment of a person who has never committed any crime (as in the notorious case of 'Typhoid Mary' in the 1910s);[4] the identification of the ones to be isolated would sometimes require violations of civil liberties in the process (AIDS patients are a case in point);[5] and finally, compulsory hospitalizations lack medical purpose when no actual cure is available (as is continuously the case with AIDS). By these remarks I am not trying to say that quarantines are always condemnable. If by the temporary isolation of one individual many other individuals can be directly saved from serious health hazards, the use of compulsory means is sometimes no doubt legitimate. What I am saying, however, is that the promotion of general good in the medical sense is not the only ethical consideration when coercive isolation and imprisonment policies are discussed.

Vaccination and Consent

Even more complicated problems arise with regard to the legitimacy of *vaccination programmes*. Although mass inoculation is usually a very effective way to prevent dangerous and fatal diseases, it is also often the cause of a few vaccine deaths among the population, and sometimes a source of bitter ideological opposition against the public health authorities.[6]

Consider, for instance, the following case presented by John M. Last:

> Faced with the outbreak of smallpox in 1947, the public health authorities of the City of New York vaccinated about 5 million people; the human costs of this were 45 known cases of post-vaccinial encephalitis [inflammation of the brain] with four deaths – an acceptable risk, in view of the enormous benefit, the safety of the city of 8 million, but a heavy price for the victims of vaccination, and their next to kin.[7]

The problems of cases like these can be divided into questions regarding consent and questions concerning other-regarding harm. I shall first say something about the former category.

As long as the programmes are organized without coercion and force, the problems are not necessarily insurmountable: if adult citizens are sufficiently informed about the risks involved and no one actually makes them take the vaccine, they can be seen as freely and knowingly – albeit implicitly – giving their consent to the procedure. That the condition of sufficient information is seldom fulfilled in the real world should give the medical authorities something to think about, but does not refute the argument itself.

When children are concerned, the validity of the proxy consent or dissent given by parents or guardians depends on the facts of the case – whether or not the child, if inoculated, has a better chance of surviving and developing into adulthood and full autonomy than without artificial immunization. But the introduction of coercion and constraint changes the situation radically. Individuals who want to forgo the vaccination do not directly harm anyone but themselves and other dissenters, and indirect harm to other people does not under the circumstances seem unproblematical as a ground for coercion either. The threshold argument could in principle be employed to support the programmes, as society might well collapse as a result of too many refusals, but it is perhaps not quite acceptable to argue that the present 'pro-vaccinal' form of society ought to be forcefully protected, if in the future the majority of citizens came to express their support to an alternative, 'anti-vaccinal' society by refusing the offered shot.

Vaccination and Harm

Regardless of the difficulties of vaccination programmes, it is not clear that the authorities would be in the right even if they decided not to inoculate the population. A rough-and-ready utilitarian calculation shows that if the public health officials of New York had chosen *not* to vaccinate the inhabitants of the city, thousands of people would have lost their lives. As the immunization programme itself only caused four deaths, the greater evil would obviously have been its absence. Thus, comparing evils, organizing the vaccination programme was the right thing to do.

There are objections to the rough-and-ready utilitarian type of thinking, most notably the claim that individuals have rights which should not be violated by the public authorities. According to this line of argument, the welfare of the majority ought not to be promoted on utilitarian grounds, because the policy would fail to respect the rights of the dissenting minority. But this view is, I think, mistaken on the simple ground that there are rights on both sides of the vaccination issue. The ones victimized by the New York smallpox immunization did, of course, have a right to be healthy and continue living. But so did the eight million inhabitants of New York who would have been at risk had the programme not been set in motion. And what could be more concrete, in the ethical sense, than the individual rights of those millions of human beings? It is obvious, when seen from this angle, that whatever the authorities had decided to do, the rights of some people would have been violated. Therefore it is probably safe to assume that the rough-and-ready utilitarian calculation which does not have universal validity could, nevertheless, have been employed to justify the decision of the New York City authorities.[8]

Persuasion

One of the methods frequently used by medical authorities to persuade people into cooperation in matters such as taking a vaccination, is the *offering of rewards*. The bait may be anything from food and medical equipment to lollipops for children, but the ethical framework remains largely the same in all situations. If what the authorities 'offer' as a reward for compliance is something that in the moral sense already belongs to the people and seems essential to their survival, the authorities are wrongfully taking advantage of the coercive situation they have themselves created, and their behaviour should be condemned.

On the other hand, if the offers presented are genuine – that is, if the goods do not morally belong to the people and are not needed quite that badly – then there is no denying that the authorities are acting in a legitimate manner. The difficulty in the latter case is, however, that offers which are not made under coercive circumstances are probably not, from the official point of view, tempting enough.

Water and Waste

Preventive measures which influence the population as a whole even more clearly than vaccinations and quarantines do, include the *installation of plumbing* and the *fluoridation of drinking water*. These societal practices are quite pervasive in the sense that if they are effected by the public authorities, practically everyone living in an industrialized society will have to face them in one form or another. The individual can, in a manner of speaking, freely decide whether or not to utilize the plumbing or to drink fluoridated water, but the pipes and the fluoride nevertheless influence one's daily routines – a refusal to drink 'official' water, for instance, would force city dwellers into buying all their drinking water from the supermarket.

These constraints, brought about in the name of general hygiene and the reduction of tooth decay, have most often been regarded as instances of paternalism, since the best interest of the population obviously is at stake here. This interpretation would, however, presuppose that public health authorities ought to be seen as benevolent physicians who are doing all in their power to 'cure' a sick community or to prevent it from catching unpleasant diseases. And the problem with this presupposition is that, according to their professional ethical codes as well as more general moral principles, doctors usually have no right to act as distributive agents – which is what the authorities of preventive medicine frequently do by removing illnesses from one part of the population (in the issue at hand, the majority developing stronger teeth) at the expense of another part (the minority developing fluoride-related diseases).

In fact, the actual justification of fluoridation and plumbing comes from other quarters, namely from the requirements of democracy and social justice. If the majority of citizens in a democratic country prefer plumbing and fluoridated drinking water to more 'natural' conditions, and express this preference through the appropriate political procedures, respect for majority rule implies, prima facie, that the opposing minority will also have to comply to the decision and, for their own part, suffer its consequences.

Exceptions to the rule are possible, of course, if the human rights of the minority would otherwise be violated, but this is hardly the case with plumbing and fluoridation: pipes presumably do not harm anybody, and although fluoride may statistically increase morbidity in the long run, this does not amount to a violation of human rights as long as there is no legal obligation to drink the 'official water'. However, if the authorities of a given country are *not* justified in putting chemicals in the drinking water, this is because they have not kept the alternatives available widely enough among the population.

Anti-smoking Policies

The methods of medical prevention introduced thus far have all been designed to make people do something that they would not do by themselves. Regulations concerning *drugs and intoxicating substances*, in their turn, usually work in the opposite direction: the purpose of the sanctions is to prevent or deter people from doing what they would or could have done had not the sanctions been set up and enforced.

Public *anti-smoking policies* provide a good illustration of the fact that most regulation related to intoxicating substances is, from the viewpoint of freedom and autonomy, unproblematic – the rights and wrongs of smoking control most often have to do with other-regarding harm and justice rather than strong paternalism.[9] Let me use as my example Finland – the country which since the enactment of the first Tobacco Act in 1976 has possessed one of the strictest legal regulations in the Western world concerning tobacco production, marketing and consumption. Based on the 1976 law, the official Finnish anti-smoking policy consisted during the late 1970s and all through the 1980s of three major categories, namely health education, price policy, and restrictions on marketing and smoking.[10] By examining these more closely one can see where the true ethical weight of the different control policies lies.

Health education in schools and via the mass media does not create even initial problems, since informing school children about the dangers of smoking belongs to the category of weak paternalism, and the spreading of information through the mass media is an instance of soft paternalism. Due to the possibility of switching channels and selecting one's reading, the general propagation of knowledge is not even prima facie autonomy-violating, and as schoolchildren do not yet possess the full adult right to self-determination, the prima facie violation of their autonomy is excused. Anti-smoking propaganda in clinics and hospitals is a different matter, because people who seek help from the physician are in an especially vulnerable position, and should not be terrorized into making less than autonomous decisions. A good demarcation line in this matter is whether the patient's symptoms indicate a tobacco-related disease or not: if they do, then informing the patient about the risks of smoking is the doctor's duty, if they do not, the patient should not be unnecessarily harassed.[11]

Price policy by differential taxation has been defended by Joel Feinberg on the grounds that smokers cumulatively and indirectly inflict harm on other people by placing on the rest of society a burden of hospitalization, medical care and lost productivity.[12] But Feinberg, and those who agree with him, tend to forget at least two considerations which may well alter the picture. First, it has nowhere been shown that smokers would actually burden the rest of society more than the average nonsmokers do – arguments like the one presented by Feinberg are mainly based on gut feeling and prejudice, and the all-important comparative element of policy judgments is entirely missing. Although smokers may die young of tobacco-related diseases, the burden they place on the national economy should at least be compared to the corresponding costs caused by nonsmokers who, surviving long after their retirement, may spend a good twenty years in idle consumption and nonproductiveness. Second, unless cigarette prices can be stratified according to the prevailing differences in income, an issue of economic injustice will arise here. Without such an arrangement, any rise in consumer prices will inevitably hit the poor harder than the rich, and assuming that smoking is a self-regarding and – for the smokers themselves – a pleasurable activity, it does not seem fair to discriminate among smokers by differences of income.

Restrictions on smoking in public premises, at schools and nurseries, in public transport and in work premises can all be justified by an appeal to the harm inflicted on other people: although the risks of 'passive smoking' have not yet been conclusively studied, it is at least clear that cigarette smoke is not healthy for children or asthmatics.[13] It is also easy to find justifications for the total ban on advertisement and sales promotion, as well as for the prohibitions against selling tobacco products to minors and – which amounts to the same thing – in unguarded slot machines. These regulations are all aimed at protecting minors from the dangers of persuasion and undue influence. Furthermore, health warnings on packages stating the tar, nicotine and carbon monoxide contents of the product can hardly be disputed on anti-paternalistic grounds, as no one is forced to read them.

Subsequently, only one of the restrictions dictated by the 1976 law in Finland can be condemned as strongly paternalistic, and this one is the ban on manufacturing and selling brands which would contain too many harmful substances measured by the standards of the Tobacco Act. There are no reliable studies indicating that 'stronger' brands would be any more dangerous to smokers than 'mild' brands, and even if there were, the prohibition, which would have to be founded on purely self-regarding grounds, would clearly be autonomy-violating. However, as the ban on 'strong' brands is the only instance of unavoidably strong paternalism in this rather extensive set of regulations, it is perhaps appropriate to conclude that smoking control is not essentially the fortress of wrongful paternalism that the tobacco industry and its lobbyists often try to make it out to be.

Illegal Drugs

Slightly different considerations are required when the control over *medicinal and narcotic drugs* instead of the traditionally accepted recreational substances is discussed. It is not the aim of public authorities to prevent people from curing themselves or others by the use of pharmaceuticals, only to protect them from any harmful side effects that many of these may, quite unexpectedly, have. To secure the protective effect, medicinals and narcotics have been divided in most Western countries into three categories: *nonprescription* drugs, which are available to anybody at request; *prescription* drugs, which can only be obtained by a doctor's written permission; and *illegal* drugs, the possession and sale of which is always prohibited and often punishable.

The possibility of compulsory withdrawal programmes for persons addicted to 'hard drugs' such as heroin, cocaine and opium raises questions concerning the persons' past and future capacity for self-determination. As far as *past autonomy* is concerned, adult drug addicts (persons who have only started the use of drugs as an adult) have been fully autonomous decision-makers once, and this fact lends certain respectability to their present choices, even if they decided to engage themselves in dangerous activities.

With regard to *future autonomy*, however, the case of the drug addict can be seen to come close to that of small children: the fragments of self-determination that presently manifest themselves in the individual's behaviour could, with proper treatment over a period of time, be transformed again into permanent and full autonomy. The question, then, is which one of the two aspects should take precedence in the matter – the choice determines whether compulsory treatment for drug addicts is justifiable.

In answering the question, it is important to note that the latter approach to the drug addict's predicament embodies two assumptions, neither of which can in fact be taken for granted.[14] First, it is assumed that drug addiction somehow renders individuals unfree and their choices nonautonomous. This idea is, no doubt, popular enough both among the general public and among medical authorities, but its validity can be questioned simply by referring to the possibility of spontaneous withdrawals from taking 'hard drugs'. If people really lost their ability to self-determination due to drug addiction, such spontaneous cases would have to be impossible – yet they exist in great numbers, and are well documented in the literature.[15] Second, those who put their faith in compulsory programmes seem to believe that it is indeed possible to forcibly 'cure people from drug addiction'. All available evidence, however, seems to indicate that unless the drug takers themselves make a self-generated decision to quit, treatments seldom have any permanent effect.[16]

The point of these remarks is that either the autonomy of drug addicts needs no saving in the first place, or that if it does, it cannot be saved unless the initiative comes from the addicts themselves. Although the actual withdrawal programme can be as constraining and coercive as need be, the patient must freely consent to the procedure to secure its success – and, consequently, its legitimacy.

If drug addicts can be as autonomous as other people, then weakly paternalistic grounds cannot justify constraints on drug sale or use, either. Moreover, as regards harm inflicted on other people, the situation is similar: the most serious drug-related threat that the authorities can point out is organized crime, but this, of course, has more to do with the illegality of the business than with any intrinsic danger emanating from the use of opium, heroin or cocaine.

The only valid reason for keeping 'hard drugs' illegal that I can think of is that where they are already banned, an uncontrolled liberalization might lead to instances of injustice which could not be tolerated. If those using intoxicating substances are mostly unemployed, uneducated youths from the lowest social classes, then a sudden free flow of drugs might kill some of them and otherwise worsen the situation for many others. But this argument stating that drugs should not be liberated at one blow is at best only a partial one. And even as such, it is an argument that cannot be supported by any reliable data, because none of these matters have been studied extensively and without prejudice.[17] The issue is complicated by many ideological and political disputes, and it sometimes seems, as two Scandinavian social scientists have put it, that illegal drugs are for most public authorities 'too good an enemy' to be lost – waging endless drug wars is often a good way to conceal really important social problems such as poverty, unemployment and the unequal distribution of civil rights.[18]

Prescription Drugs

Let me move on, however, to an apparently less dramatic case, which nevertheless raises interesting ethical questions – the case of *prescription drug laws* and their justification. Many liberal theorists have believed that weakly paternalistic grounds can be found for accepting such laws, since ordinary people do not know enough about the side effects of various medicinal drugs to make sufficiently voluntary and autonomous decisions concerning their use.[19] Other liberal theorists, notably J.S. Mill, have disagreed with this view, arguing that if 'voluntariness' and 'autonomy' are defined too strictly, many other activities besides the sale of dangerous drugs would have to be prohibited as well, in a spirit that would be quite illiberal.[20] And recently a third approach has been introduced by George W. Rainbolt, who has argued[21] that prescription drug laws are justifiable but *strongly paternalistic*.[22] If this third view is correct, prescription laws in fact constitute a counterexample against liberal views like the one I have been defending in this book, since my claim has been that strong paternalism is never justified, and that it is always illegitimate to constrain fully autonomous behaviour 'in the agent's own best interest'.

Rainbolt's argument is based on a distinction between two levels of knowledge concerning drugs, originally presented by Joel Feinberg.[23] Ordinary citizens who take drugs either for medicinal or recreational purposes do not as a rule know much about the substances as such, but they do know about their own ignorance in the matter and about the implications of this ignorance. Ordinary citizens, then, lack *first-level knowledge* about drugs, but possess relevant *metaknowledge* which, according to Rainbolt, enable them to make hazardous decisions with their 'eyes wide open', or to put the matter in more technical terms, with sufficient voluntariness and autonomy. Thus weakly paternalistic grounds cannot be employed to justify intervention, and if the laws in question are justifiable, as Rainbolt believes they are, then their ethical basis must be strongly paternalistic.

C.L. Ten criticizes Rainbolt by arguing that metaknowledge concerning one's own ignorance does not, as such, make an agent's decision's voluntary.[24] He writes:

> Very much depends on what the relevant metaknowledge is supposed to include. If all that is required is that people know that they are ignorant about drugs, then indeed we can attribute such metaknowledge to them. But metaknowledge of this kind is compatible with first-level ignorance which cancels voluntariness in risk-taking. Thus an ignorant drug-user might be unaware of the high risk that she is taking because she does not know that the drug can cause very grave harm. She does not therefore voluntarily take the risk of grave harm.[25]

Ten concludes that weak paternalism, based on concrete first-level ignorance, is what – despite the existence of the vague metaknowledge – justifies prescription laws for some drugs.[26]

As Rainbolt correctly points out in a reply, however, Ten by his comment raises the difficult issue of setting limits to (weakly) paternalistic interventions: if first-level ignorance always implied legitimate constraint, then there should be, for instance, laws prohibiting unknowledgeable persons from fixing their own car brakes.[27] Moreover, I am not entirely convinced that Ten is right in his analysis of the relationship between the two kinds of knowledge in the drug-user example. It is certainly true that an ignorant decision-maker might 'not know that the drug can cause very grave harm' – but this is only crucial if she lacks *both* the first-level knowledge *and* the metaknowledge concerning her own ignorance. The relevant metaknowledge would simply be that the agent consciously knows that she *does not know whether or not the drug in question is seriously harmful.* If she knows this, there is nothing to stop her from making relatively voluntary and autonomous choices.

Keeping these remarks in mind, it is interesting to consider one further retort that consistent 'weak' paternalists could make in defence of their own position. What they could claim, namely, is that ordinary citizens who have not had medical training do not, in fact, know about their own ignorance concerning drugs, and do not, therefore, in the real world possess the relevant metaknowledge attributed to them by Rainbolt. As this is an empirical claim, not a conceptual argument, the 'weak' paternalists are free to agree with Rainbolt's theory of metaknowledge – all that is stated is that the theory does not apply to the prevailing social reality.

There is obviously a grain of truth in this counterargument, and it is therefore quite possible that weakly paternalistic grounds could, after all, be employed to justify some prescription drug laws for potentially harmful medicinals. But granted that this is true one must, at this point, start looking for explanations: *why* is it that ordinary drug-consuming citizens do not even know that their ignorance may be fatal? One popular answer to this question is that because the variety of drugs is so great nowadays, people simply cannot master even the most elementary pharmacological questions concerning the drugs they use. But this response is, in our present context, beside the point: regardless of the variety and diversity, it is surely possible to inform people about the general risk. After all, it was not required in Mill's famous bridge example,[28] that the crosser should be given a course in construction engineering before he can be allowed to cross the river.

The only other explanation that comes readily to mind connects the legal requirement of prescriptions with the role and status of the medical profession in Western societies. Prescription drug laws are extremely important and useful to physicians, who through the power of the legal system are given the monopoly to control what drugs people use and when. This arrangement naturally opens channels for them in the direction of the medical industry as well, and it is understandable that doctors would not like to lose their key position in the presumably quite profitable prescription drug game.

But explanations of this kind are for sociologists rather than philosophers to tackle, and I must return to the conceptual issues. From this point of view, the foregoing considerations seem to imply that although prescription drug laws may at the moment be justifiable, owing to the prevailing lack of metaknowledge, it does not follow from this that the laws ought to be upheld indefinitely. Rather, the ethical implication is that people ought to be provided with health education and drug information so that they could become masters of their own lives in using drugs as well as in accepting or refusing other treatments.

Incidentally, this latter point also means that Rainbolt is ultimately more correct than his critic Ten on the issue of metaknowledge and its significance. Fortunately, however, it cannot be inferred from this that Rainbolt is right in his other claim: he does not actually prove the legitimacy of prescription drug laws in his article, and thus his argument concerning the moral status of strong paternalism remains unsubstantiated. Consequently, I am left free to conclude that strong paternalism never provides valid grounds for restricting people's liberty and violating their autonomy 'in their own best interest'.

Notes

Parts of this chapter have been strongly influenced by Heta Häyry and Matti Häyry, 'Utilitarianism, human rights and the redistribution of health through preventive medical measures', *Journal of Applied Philosophy* **6**: 43–51; and Heta Häyry, Matti Häyry and Sakari Karjalainen, 'Paternalism and Finnish anti-smoking policy', *Social Science and Medicine* **28**: 293–297. My thanks are due to Dr Mark Shackleton, Lecturer in English, University of Helsinki, for checking my English.

1   J. Feinberg, *Harm to Self* (Oxford and New York: Oxford University Press, 1986), pp. 21–23.

2   D. Mayo, 'AIDS, quarantines, and non-compliant positives', in D. VanDeVeer and C. Pierce (eds), *AIDS: Ethics and Public Policy* (Belmont, Cal.: Wadsworth, 1988); M. Häyry and H. Häyry, 'AIDS, society and morality – A philosophical survey', *Philosophia* **19** (1989): 331–361.

3   See, e.g., T.S. Szasz, *The Manufacture of Madness: A Comparative Study of the Inquisition and the Mental Health Movement* (London: Routledge & Kegan Paul, 1971), pp. 182 ff., on 'masturbatory insanity' as an alleged cause of hereditary diseases and ground for isolation of the 'patient' in a madhouse.

4   Mary Mallon, a.k.a. 'Typhoid Mary', was an Irish-born cook who in her work in New York accidentally infected several people with typhoid fever. In 1925 she was imprisoned indefinitely, because the authorities wanted to protect the general public from the innocent threat posed by her cooking. She died 23 years later, still imprisoned, without ever having committed a punishable crime.

5   R.D. Mohr, 'AIDS, gays and state coercion', *Bioethics* **1** (1987): 35–50; Mayo 1988.

6   J.M. Last, *Public Health and Human Ecology* (Ottawa: Appleton & Lange, 1987), p. 354.

7   Last 1987, p. 354.

8   This theme has been developed further in the article on utilitarianism and human rights mentioned in the beginning of the notes to this chapter.

9   The question in the Finnish context has been discussed in more detail in the article on smoking policy mentioned in the beginning of the notes to this chapter.

10   K. Leppo, and H. Vertio, 'Smoking control in Finland: A case study in policy formulation and implementation', *Health Promotion* **1** (1986): 5-16. Leppo and Vertio present, as a matter of fact, a fourth category as well: (4) research, planning and evaluation. But since this set of activities is obviously subsidiary to the first three groups, I shall not examine it separately. The same applies, incidentally, to a subactivity within the third category, namely quality control.

11   This demarcation line was suggested to me by Dr Sakari Karjalainen.

12   J. Feinberg, *Harm to Others* (Oxford and New York: Oxford University Press, 1984), pp. 23-25.

13   E. O'Connel and G.B. Logan, 'Parental smoking in childhood asthma', *Annales of Allergy* **32** (1974): 142-145; I.B. Tager, S.T. Weiss, B. Rosnerand and F.E. Speizer, 'Effect of parental cigarette smoking on the pulmanory function of children', *American Journal of Epidemiology* **110** (1979): 15-26; A. Knight, and A.B. Breslin, 'Passive cigarette smoking and patients with asthma', *Medical Journal of Australia* **142** (1985): 194-195.

14   G. Graham, 'Drugs, freedom and harm', in C. Peden and J.K. Roth (eds), *Rights, Justice, and Community* (Lewiston, Queenston and Lampeter: The Edwin Mellen Press, 1992).

15   S. Caplin, and S. Woodward, *Drugwatch: Just say No!* (London, 1986), p. 59.

16   Caplin and Woodward 1986, p. 74; T. Stewart, *The Heroin Users*, (London, 1987), ch. 7.

17   A good philosophical survey of problems related to 'hard drugs' is Graham 1992.

18   N. Christie, and K. Bruun, *Den gode fiende (The Good Enemy*, in Norwegian) (Oslo: Universitetsforlaget, 1985).

19   Feinberg 1986, pp. 127-133; C.L. Ten, 'Paternalism and levels of knowledge: A comment on Rainbolt', *Bioethics* **3** (1989): 135-139.

20   J.S. Mill, *On Liberty* (1859), reprinted in R. Wollheim (ed.), *Three Essays* (Oxford: Oxford University Press, 1975), pp. 118-119; R.J. Arneson, 'Mill versus paternalism', *Ethics* **90** (1980): 471-489, p. 482.

21   G.W. Rainbolt, 'Prescription drug laws: justified hard paternalism', *Bioethics* **3** (1989a): 45-58.

22   To be exact, Rainbolt discusses 'hard paternalism' here, following Feinberg's later terminology and definitions, but his argument can equally well be directed against 'strong paternalism' in the sense I have defined it in chapter 3 above.

23   Rainbolt 1989a, pp. 50 ff.; Feinberg 1986, p. 161.

24   Ten 1989.

25   Ten 1989, p. 136.

26   Ten 1989, pp. 138–139.

27   G.W. Rainbolt, 'Justified hard paternalism: A response to Ten', *Bioethics* **3** (1989b): 140–141; Rainbolt 1989a, pp. 52–53.

28   Mill 1859, p. 118. More about the example in chapter 2 above.

6 Aids, Discrimination and Legal Restrictions

When the acquired immune deficiency syndrome, AIDS, was first discovered, it was seen predominantly as a gay problem. Initially, in 1981, it was believed that the disease only spread through male homosexual intercourse. Later it was found out that blood transfusions and blood contact in general are also possible sources of human immunodeficiency virus, or HIV, infection. But even after the first genuinely heterosexual chains of infection were reported, it still seemed to many people that the problem of AIDS is a gay problem. Although it was clear at this stage that not only male homosexuals with certain habits were at risk, it was still the credo that all proper steps taken to fight the disease had something to do with discriminating against homosexuals or passing restrictive legislation directed against behaviour which was regarded as dangerous or indecent.

But all this was, or at least should have been, radically changed by 1986. It was predicted in and after the Second International Conference on AIDS, arranged in Paris, June 1986, that AIDS will seriously threaten the heterosexual population in the near future in the Western countries if the spread of the HIV cannot be effectively controlled. Whatever the accuracy of the prediction, AIDS should have ceased to be a problem merely for homosexuals at that time. On one hand, it had by then become clear that gay men are not the only ones who have to worry about the risk of infection. And on the other, it is of no use to discriminate against one minority group when the disease that should be suppressed is not restriced to that one group.

During the last decade, however, the attitudes concerning AIDS have in many places remained similar to the first reactions experienced in the beginning of the 1980s. I shall, in this chapter, examine and refute some of the explanations and justifications given in defence of discriminatory and legally restrictive practices and regulations.

The Logic of Discrimination

In attitudes and behaviour towards people who are known to be infected with HIV, two moral codes, utilitarianism and egoism, collide. According to utilitarian thinking, what people do should be determined by calculations concerning the good of all, whereas the egoistic code allows people to restrict their attention solely to their own good, or the good of those near them. There are good theoretical as well as practical grounds for preferring, in general, utilitarianism to egoism. But since even the good of all may presuppose that individuals and groups are allowed to have a certain sphere of immunity of their own, it is not wise to jump to conclusions. Let me study, instead, the situation itself a little more closely.

The women and men in the street often appear to be quite utilitarian when they judge the behaviour and interests of other people. If, for instance, doctors and nurses announced that it is their right to refuse to treat AIDS patients, vociferous objections would, no doubt, be heard. Medical personnel are supposed to work for the good of all their patients, and any attempt at discrimination according to sex, skin colour, religion or medical condition is automatically ruled out.

But there is a radical change in attitudes when the problem is brought near enough to the ordinary citizen. Should children infected with HIV be allowed to go to the same school as noninfected children? What about hiring a person with AIDS at an office? Put face to face with questions like these, the ordinary citizen immediately starts producing excuses and explanations, typically claiming that her family is, in fact, unlike any other family in certain relevant respects. 'Our children are used to rough games; they could bite an AIDS child and become infected through blood contact.' Or, 'I myself have such a weak heart; I couldn't bear the extra stress caused by a coworker with AIDS'.

It is not altogether clear whether excuses like these reflect ill-concealed egoism or misinformed utilitarianism or a mixture of both. But one thing is clear: if and when people use utilitarian arguments when they judge other people's behaviour, they should accept that the same line of argument can also be applied to their own actions. If they do not accept this, the only kind of moral theory open to them is egoism as determined by the principle 'I have the right to pursue my own good, even at the expense of the good of all, but all other people have a duty to pursue the good of all, even at the expense of their own good'. Unlike some other forms of ethical egoism, this particular form lacks one of the basic qualities every moral theory must have: its precepts are not universalizable. 'I' cannot accept that anyone else acts according to this theory, since it would contradict my possibility of employing it. And it is the core of ethical theories that they should apply in the same way to all relevantly similar people.[1]

What the person in the street is left with, at this point, is utilitarian argumentation. There are three ways to argue in favour of discrimination within this framework, but not one of them leads to the desired result.

Firstly, it could be claimed that we and our children really do differ from all other people in a respect that makes us markedly more vulnerable to the attacks of HIV infection than others are. But, apart from a few exceptions, all people are in exactly the same position with regard to acquiring HIV infection from a schoolmate or a colleague. There are no significant differences between individuals in this matter. Contact with the body fluids of already infected persons always carries a risk of contagion, and this risk has little to do with who and what we are in other respects.

Secondly, although we all face the same risk of infection if we are exposed to the virus, perhaps the risk is so grave that all noninfected people have a right to discriminate against the infected. Perhaps the dissident doctors and nurses are ultimately right: maybe it is, after all, perfectly acceptable that they refuse to treat potential AIDS patients. Perhaps HIV-infected people are so dangerous that the only thing we can do to protect ourselves is to isolate them, as suggested by some overtly cautious officials in the 1980s.[2] This line of argument, however, grossly contradicts the facts. HIV does not spread in everyday social intercourse, and the possibility of being bitten or raped by an HIV-infected person at school or at work is, most probably, slimmer than the risk of, say, being fatally hit by a car. But as traffic accidents are reduced by taking precautions and giving information, not by discriminating against car owners, the same peaceful procedures should be utilized in preventing AIDS-related accidents in everyday situations.

Thirdly, in addition to these subjective and supposedly objective attempts to justify discrimination, an intersubjective justification is, in principle, possible. Although victims of HIV do not spread their infection in ordinary social life, they can, from a religious or moralistic point of view, be considered bad and sinful persons who 'get what they deserve'.[3] By merely existing they offend the moral values of large groups of people. This is why many people from these latter groups think that discrimination against them is acceptable.

The Lure of Legal Moralism

Let me take a closer look at the intersubjective arguments in connection with a specific form of discrimination: the legal restriction of personal choices.

The philosophical concepts associated with the matter are *legal moralism* and *harm to others*.

According to legal moralism, sin should be legally punished and in this way morality should be enforced for morality's sake.[4] The most significant requirements of legal moralism regarding the AIDS issue are the demands to prohibit by law premarital sexual relationships, extramarital relationships, 'perversions' in marital sexual life, homosexual behaviour, prostitution, and the misuse of intravenous drugs. Many people have thought that such prohibitions, if properly enforced, would have a considerable impact on the spread of sexually transmissible diseases, including AIDS. (This, of course, is only a theoretical list, and has not to my knowledge been presented as such. But the accuracy of the list is not the point here. The prohibition of all these things is, in any case, the ultimate aim of many influential religious and conservative groups.)

Legal moralism is, in itself, a rather problematic doctrine. 'Sin' and 'morality for morality's sake' only exist in people's minds and in their shared beliefs and attitudes. But if people are free to choose their own actions and norms – as the legal moralist believes they are – then these things are apt to vary not only among different groups of people but also during different periods of time. Furthermore, in modern Western cultures we tend to have many differing opinions concerning sin and morality for morality's sake even within one society or one nation. How do we know, then, which opinion is the right one, or whether, indeed, there *is* a right one?

Since legal moralists themselves are nowadays well aware of the fact that terms like 'sin' and 'morality for morality's sake' mean different things to different people, they have, for lay audiences, slightly altered their own line of argument. Enforcing morality as such is, they can now say, the right thing to do because morality as such is something that maintains the fabric of society, and provides the basis for the meaningful pursuit of happiness. If morality as such – as 'we' understand it – is not regarded as an absolute value any more, 'our' society will collapse and 'we' shall be left with no real basis for our efforts. Anarchy does not provide the firm ground that we need to build our lives firmly on.

This is, however, the right argument applied to the wrong thing. It may be true that we need laws, order, and morality as such in order to pursue personal happiness. But as far as the argument goes, any moderately reasonable set of laws and moral codes will do. It would only be a matter of education to teach future generations to accept, say, the whole variety of hetero as well as homosexual activities. In any case, the legal prohibition of these activities cannot be justified by appeals to legal moralism.

What about justifying legal restrictions by referring to the harm inflicted on other people by 'immoral' behaviour? This brings the discussion back to the supposedly objective attempts to justify discrimination, although the discrimination would, this time, be directed against larger groups of people. It could be argued that since liberal sex habits, homosexual behaviour, prostitution, and intravenous drug use are likely to spread AIDS and other sexually transmissible diseases, they should be prohibited and severely sanctioned so as to protect all the prospective victims of these diseases. And it seems that this kind of argument is based on a plausible normative premise. If serious harm to others can be prevented by restricting dangerous behaviour, it should, no doubt, be done. However, it is not the normative premise that plays the central role in the argument. The real problem emerges from the falsehood of the factual premise.

Although liberal sex habits, prostitution, and drug use most probably help certain diseases to spread, the spread cannot be suppressed by legal sanctions. There are two kinds of activities here, and neither of them is likely to be affected by restrictive laws. Firstly, whether one engages in 'dangerous' sex or not is generally considered to be a strictly personal matter, not a matter for the law. There are two historical examples that show quite clearly the futility, even danger, of trying to force people to change their behaviour in such matters. Prohibition in the United States and in some European countries is the patent Western example of a well-meaning yet ill-fated piece of legal regulation. On the other hand, there have been, and in some cases still are, laws that forbid all kinds of sex save intramarital heterosexual intercourse in the missionary position. Naturally enough, these laws have not made any marked difference on what people do in the privacy of their bedrooms or wherever they practice sex.

Secondly, although things like prostitution and the misuse of drugs almost always include elements that cannot be considered strictly personal, their legal prohibition in most countries has not really put an end to them. On the contrary, what has been achieved by restrictive laws is that organized crime has taken over these branches of business, and lacking governmental control this has created violence and disorder in every major city in the Western world. Instead of wasting their efforts in planning additional constraints, authorities should, perhaps, rather think about annulling at least some parts of the existing regulation.

Re-criminalizing homosexuality is yet another issue. There is evidence[5] to the effect that it is the *de*criminalization of homosexual behaviour that has had a positive impact on preventing the spread of sexually transmissible diseases, not the reenforcement of legal restrictions. Restrictive laws seem to press homosexuals into a number of anonymous contacts instead of stable relationships. And it is in these anonymous contacts that the danger of fatal epidemics lies. In the absence of legal and social pressures, on the other hand, homosexual men are more apt to create 'safe' permanent relationships with each other.

The only expected positive effect of legal restrictions concerning personal sex matters is, in the last analysis, the relief some conscientious people with traditional views would experience. But this is hardly enough to outweigh the negative effects: the harm inflicted on individuals by persecuting them because of their sexual drives, and the possible harm inflicted on society by indirectly encouraging illegal activities. Not only are the disutilities quantitatively greater than the expected utilities, but they are qualitatively of a higher order as well. Even if a classical utilitarian calculation showed that legal moralists, being superior in numbers, experience, on the whole, more pleasure than gays and other members of suppressed groups feel pain, the laws would still be unjust. This is because rational, well-informed people do not lose their opportunities to lead happy lives just because they know that somebody out there is 'sinning'. However, being deprived of the possibility of having a satisfactory and harmless sex life, gays and other members of oppressed minorities do lose the opportunity to lead happy lives if restrictive laws are established. And happiness, rather than the aggregate pleasure, is what counts in deciding whether or not a given course of action, or a given set of laws, is the right one.

It seems, then, that discrimination and legal sex restrictions are not the way to fight AIDS. They do not suppress the spread of the disease, but they do cause unhappiness to HIV-infected persons, to homosexuals, and to people who prefer many sex partners. In addition, they can actually help the spread of AIDS: if people know that HIV infection is a punishable thing to have, they dare not go to the tests, and even if they have themselves tested and the result is positive, they can conceal the result from other people. In such circumstances many people may be infected quite unnecessarily, say, because carriers of the virus are too afraid of revealing themselves to insist on the use of a condom in sexual intercourse.

Questions in HIV Testing

Testing for HIV antibodies has been one of the most contentious issues in the AIDS debate since a reliable test method was developed in 1984.[6] Public opinion has during the past decade gradually shifted from the initial demands to test compulsorily all homosexuals to the tacit acceptance of voluntary testing for the general public and routine semi-mandatory testing for those whose behaviour is supposed to put them in a high-risk bracket. In the debate, no one actually denies the importance of attaining epidemiological knowledge concerning the spread of AIDS, and very few find anonymous screening – if *total* anonymity can be guaranteed – in the hospitals or in some such places morally offensive. The real issues are whether or not patients have given their informed consent to test, and when should a positive result be disclosed, for one reason or another, to the tested themselves or to some other party.

The most restrictive policy option, mandatory screening for HIV, has been explicitly advocated only by a handful of public authorities and physicians, and even these have often used euphemistic expressions like 'required testing' to soften their message. Yet there is, in principle, a perfect justification for mandatory measures – an appeal to the rights of the non-infected. Although a person who does not wish to know her or his HIV antibody status does have a prima facie right not to be told, this right, based on respect towards the person's autonomy, can be overridden by the right of her or his sexual partners not to contract the deadly virus in case the person happens to be a carrier, but does not take precautions because of being unaware of her or his own infectivity.

The problem with this justification is, however, that it contains an important factual premise which is not inevitably tenable. As I have already shown in the above that legal restrictions are not the answer to questions evoked by AIDS, other people's rights will be protected only if those infected with HIV voluntarily change their patterns of sexual behaviour along with the knowledge of the infection. But as long as known HIV carriers have to face varying degrees of discrimination, fear, and moral contempt from their fellow human beings, this factual premise does not necessarily hold, and the argument remains materially invalid.

The first step in the moderate direction is to advocate routine instead of mandatory testing. This means, roughly, that certain specified groups – for instance, everybody who enters hospital or is examined by a doctor or serves in the army, all pregnant women, all convicted drug addicts, all those who have other sexually transmissible diseases, and all those travellers who return home from areas where the prevalence of AIDS is high – would be automatically tested on convenient occasions, the motive for the procedure being that the people health authorities would like to see tested do not test themselves voluntarily, due to fear of stigmatization. However, whereas mandatory testing can be performed even against the person's expressed wishes, this is not the case with routine testing. In the latter case, the patient's consent is implicitly assumed until she or he explicitly denies it: *implied consent* is the justification of routine testing against claims of violations of people's privacy or autonomy.

Brenda Almond, for instance, has argued in favour of this kind of view, stating that since 'precisely the people it is necessary to reach' most probably evade voluntary testing, and since, on the other hand, it is also important 'to ensure that people would not forego essential treatment through reluctance to be [mandatorily] tested', a compromise should be found between the extremes.[7] Her own suggestion is that blood taken for other purposes ought to be available for HIV as well as other kinds of additional testing, and that the antibody status of patients with sexually transmissible diseases should be routinely checked, 'unless a patient specifically requests that this should not be done'.[8]

But implied consent is not as unproblematic an issue as those relying on it would like to believe. There was a heated debate on the matter among the official representatives of the British Medical Association as early as the autumn of 1987, and the medicolegal conclusion of the discussion was that English law at least would strongly condemn any attempts from the side of physicians to treat or test their patients without the patients' genuine, informed and explicit consent.[9] The ethically as well as legally noteworthy reason for this condemnation was that although 'the patient does not need to be told everything' in every medical situation, she or he must, nevertheless, 'understand the nature of the procedure the doctor proposes to carry out and the real risks attached'.[10] Since the very real risks of suddenly and without warning becoming aware of one's HIV positivity range from depression to suicide, and since there is no known cure for the disease which may develop, informed consent is obviously of utmost importance in HIV testing. And in order to receive the patients' informed consent the doctor should, in fact, provide them with 'pre-test counselling', instead of trying not to mention even the possibility of the 'routine' test in the fear that they might otherwise explicitly refuse to give their permission to its performance.

The drastic solution would then, be that HIV testing is acceptable only if a person voluntarily and deliberately expresses the wish to be tested, *and* even then only after a session of intensive pre-test counselling by experts in medical, psychological, and social matters. What I think, however, is that either one of the conditions separately suffices to justify a decision to test a person's HIV antibody status. It would be ethically almost as dubious as mandatory screening to deny people the test on the grounds that they refuse to take part in serious counselling beforehand, and thus render themselves incapable of giving *informed* consent to the procedure.

Some of those who profess only voluntary measures would agree with me that being fully informed cannot be a necessary condition for testing in case a person herself or himself initiates the process and freely consents to it. But many of them would probably hold that the relevance of explicit consent still makes a difference - that it at least automatically outlaws any attempts to set up a routine testing programme. If, however, testing is important in the prevention of the spread of AIDS, and if its importance is taken as seriously as the undeniable significance of consent, it seems that whatever the difficulties in contemporary medical practice or social life, authorities ought to do their best to combine the two interests.

The solution, in principle at least, would be routinely testing everybody who enters a hospital or seeks the help of a physician *and* genuinely consents to be tested after receiving adequate information. Admittedly this could, at the moment, be difficult to realize - doctors ought to be better trained in counselling, and besides, they do not always have the time to involve themselves in such activity. But the more efficient the general information campaigns have become during the years, the easier it has become for doctors to achieve patients' informed consent - or dissent - to HIV testing. Although HIV testing does differ from most standard medical procedures in important respects, it is surely not unique enough to require permanent special arrangements.

What is required in the discussion concerning HIV and AIDS is that public health authorities understand both the need of the infected to live as normally as possible *and* the desire of the others not to be infected in the first place.[11]

Notes

Early versions of parts of this chapter have been published as Heta Häyry and Matti Häyry, 'AIDS now', *Bioethics* 1 (1987): 339-356; and Matti Häyry and Heta Häyry, 'AIDS, society and morality - A philosophical survey', *Philosophia* 19 (1989): 331-361. My thanks are due to Dr Mark Shackleton, Lecturer in English, University of Helsinki, for checking my English.

1   See, e.g., R.M. Hare, *Moral Thinking: Its Levels, Method and Point* (Oxford: Clarendon Press, 1981), pp. 108-116. Cf. J. Rawls, *A Theory of Justice*, Oxford, Oxford University Press 1972, p. 132; R.B. Brandt, *A Theory of the Good and the Right*, Oxford, Clarendon Press 1979, pp. 229-230; P. Singer, *Practical Ethics*, Cambridge, Cambridge University Press 1979, pp. 10-13.

2   Even if this argument were valid, there would be serious difficulties. Whom exactly should we isolate, or quarantine? All persons with AIDS? This would leave the majority of HIV infected and infectious people free to spread the

disease. All those who have HIV sero-positive test results? A question of room and expenses arises: if there are millions of people infected by HIV in the world and all of them were quarantined for life, where could the authorities put them? These things are lucidly discussed by D.J. Mayo, 'AIDS, quarantines, and non-compliant positives', in D. VanDeVeer and C. Pierce (eds), *AIDS: Ethics and Social Policy* (Belmont, Cal.: Wadsworth, 1988).

3   See, e.g., R.D. Mohr, 'AIDS, gays and state coercion', *Bioethics* **1** (1987): 35-50, p. 36 n. 3.

4   I have analyzed the nature and attempted justifications of legal moralism in *The Limits of Medical Paternalism* (London and New York: Routledge, 1991), ch. 4.

5   K. Sinclair and M. Ross, 'Consequences of decriminalisation of homosexuality: a study of two Australian States', *Journal of Homosexuality* **12** (1986): 119-127.

6   As Sirkka-Liisa Valle writes: 'There are three major ways of identifying an HIV-infected individual: First, by detecting an immune response in the host by measuring the anti-HIV antibodies; Second, by detecting circulating HIV antigen; And third, by isolating the virus.' (*Predisposing Factors and Early Characteristics of Human Immunodeficiency Virus (HIV) Infection in a Cohort of Homosexual Men in Finland*, Helsinki: University Press, 1987, p. 13.) Since the test ordinarily used for detecting anti-HIV antibodies 'is suspectible to false-positive reactions', more accurate measures are used to confirm the results. When I refer to HIV testing here, I we mean antibody testing confirmed by other modes of identifying the infection.

7   B. Almond, 'AIDS and international ethics', *Ethics & International Affairs* **2** (1988): 139-154, p. 149.

8   Almond 1988, p. 149.

9   C. Dyer, 'Testing for HIV: the medicolegal view', *British Medical Journal* **295** (1987): 871-872; M. Sherrad and I. Gatt, 'Human immunodeficiency virus (HIV) antibody testing', *British Medical Journal* **295** (1987): 911-912; 'No HIV testing without consent, say lawyers', *British Medical Journal* **295** (1987): 936-937.

10   Dyer 1987, p. 872.

11   This dual requirement has been well analysed in J. Harris and C. Erin, 'AIDS: ethics, justice and social policy', *Journal of Applied Philosophy* **10** (1993): 165-173.

7 Does Democratic Might Make Right in Health Care Policy-making?

In a scene of *A Woman of No Importance* where politics and health are conversed Oscar Wilde lets the persons of the play make many observations which are pertinent to the themes of this book, namely the questions of life, liberty and decision-making in health care. Lady Hunstanton starts the discussion by commenting upon the effects of democracy:

> Politics are in a sad way, everywhere, I am told. They certainly are in England. Dear Mr. Cardew is ruining the country. I wonder Mrs. Cardew allows him. I am sure, Lord Illingworth, you don't think that uneducated people should be allowed to have votes?[1]

To which Lord Illingworth replies:

> I think they are the only people who should.[2]

Having thus given the claim to political expertise to the uneducated Lord Illingworth, however, responding to Kelvil's question, limits the validity of this claim to the uneducated of his own class. The exchange proceeds as follows:

> KELVIL: May I ask, Lord Illingworth, if you regard the House of Lords as a better institution than the House of Commons?
> LORD ILLINGWORTH: A much better institution, of course. We in the House of Lords are never in touch with public opinion. That makes us a civilised body.[3]

If Lord Illingworth's elitism tends to seem inpalatable to the democratic minds of today, it is useful to remember the kind of public opinion he is referring to. Immediately preceeding the line I have just quoted he criticizes the concept of health prevailing in the society of his day:

Silliest word in our language, [health] and one knows so well the popular idea of health. The English country gentleman galloping after a fox – the unspeakable in full pursuit of the uneatable.[4]

Health and social policies also enter the discussion more directly, when Lady Hunstanton takes up Lord Illingworth's idea of amusing the poor:

Certainly, a great deal may be done by means of cheap entertainments, as you say, Lord Illingworth. Dear Dr. Daubeny, our rector here, provides, with the assistance of his curates, really admirable recreations for the poor during the winter. And much good may be done by means of a magic lantern, or a missionary, or some popular amusement of that kind.[5]

A discordant voice is heard when Lady Caroline joins the conversation, and retorts:

I am not at all in favour of amusements for the poor, Jane. Blankets and coals are sufficient. There is too much love of pleasure among the upper classes as it is. Health is what we want in modern life. The tone is not healthy, not healthy at all.[6]

To which Lord Illingworth presents his fox-hunt definition of health, and the discussion floats to other topics.

The Problem

In the passages that I have just quoted Oscar Wilde manages to touch most of the themes that are important to public decision-making and the role of moral expertise in health care. The questions his persons pose include: What is health? What is health care policy? What kind of health care policy should be preferred? Who gets to make these policies? And should popular opinion be heard, or respected, or obeyed, in health care policy-making? The last-mentioned question is the one that I intend to answer, to the best of my abilities, in this chapter.

The question as expressed by the title of the chapter is: Does democratic might make right? By the term 'democratic' I refer to attitudes and practices favouring democracy, and by 'democracy' mainly some kind of government by the people, especially a rule of the majority. So my title really asks:

Does the fact that health care policymakers favour in their work the rule of the majority, or the government of the people more generally, make their decisions morally correct, or legitimate, or justifiable?

Or, to put the matter in terms of the broader topic of moral expertise in health care in general:

Are the people the moral experts in health care policy-making, and if they are, in what sense?

To answer these questions I shall have to begin by examining what forms the policy of favouring democracy can assume within different ideologies and philosophical theories.

Contemporary Moral and Political Philosophies: an Outline

There are two main dividing lines between the most important twentieth-century normative theories of moral and political philosophy. The first distinction concerns the nature of human freedom. Those who believe that freedom means the absence of restrictions have been said to uphold a *negative concept of liberty*, while those who believe that freedom means the presence of certain rationally, emotionally, politically or morally defensible restrictions have been labelled as supporters of a *positive concept of liberty*.[7]

The second distinction concerns the existence and legitimacy of a category of rights which can be called 'positive claim-rights'. These are rights which entitle their bearers to the positive help of others in situations where they cannot cope with matters by themselves. One set of moral and political philosophers hold that positive claim-rights can only be valid in situations where they can be supported by *prior contracts, covenants, promises, natural hierarchies between individuals, or their special relationships with each other*. Thus I can have the right that you buy me an ice cream on the grounds that I bought you one yesterday and you promised to buy me one today, or because I belong to the class of people who are – for reasons that only philosophers of the right persuasion can specify – universally entitled to free ice creams, or because I am your aunt or your niece and aunts and nieces should be bought ice creams whenever they want them.

Another set of philosophers argue that while all these reasons can under certain circumstances be at least partly legitimate, there is a further reason which alone can make positive claim-rights truly valid, namely *need*. In the context of my example, if I am starving and you are not, and if you can feed me with your ice cream, then you have a duty to do so, and I have a positive right that corresponds to your duty. The situation can, of course, be more complicated – for instance, if there are several people who are starving and you can only help one of them, you have no automatic obligation to choose me. But what the champions of the need principle would maintain is that, say, if my vital needs are in conflict with your niece's 'natural', family-based entitlement to the ice cream, then my needs should be seen as the overriding moral consideration in the case.[8]

When the two distinctions are crossed, the result can be presented in the schematic form seen in Figure 7.1.

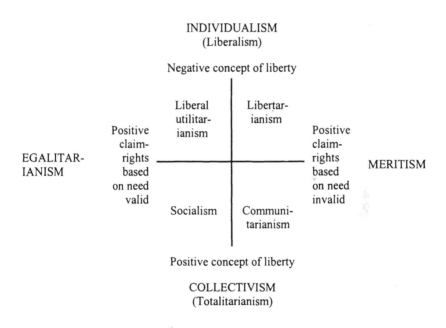

INDIVIDUALISM
(Liberalism)

Negative concept of liberty

	Liberal utilitarianism	Libertarianism	
EGALITARIANISM	Positive claim-rights based on need valid		Positive claim-rights based on need invalid	MERITISM
	Socialism	Communitarianism	

Positive concept of liberty

COLLECTIVISM
(Totalitarianism)

Figure 7.1   Contemporary moral and political theories

The moral and political philosophies that uphold the negative concept of liberty can be classified under the labels 'individualism' and – with some hesitation – 'liberalism'. The hesitation stems from the fact that traditional deontological moralists like Immanuel Kant are nowadays often counted among liberal thinkers, although theories like his cannot fully accomodate the negative concept of liberty. The supporters of the positive concept of liberty, in their turn, place collectives before individuals, and sometimes also the totality – that is, the state or society as a whole – before its parts or members. The use of the epithets 'collectivism' and 'totalitarianism' is, therefore, justified.

When positive claim-rights are not based on needs, they must be based on 'natural' distinctions, status differences, deserts or other kinds of inborn or acquired merits – this is why I have coined the phrase 'meritism' for the theories on the right-hand side of the figure. When, on the other hand, positive claim-rights *are* based on needs, everybody's dues are measured equally according to need – thus 'egalitarianism' is an apt name for the views depicted on the left.

Libertarian and Socialist Thinking

The four views I have singled out in the figure – libertarianism, socialism, communitarianism and liberal utilitarianism – are examples of modern theories which can be found in the opposite ends of the ideological continuums. All these doctrines can be democratic in their own ways, but the content of the principle of 'democracy' varies considerably from one theory to another.

According to *libertarian* thinking, the correct idea of democracy is that individuals appoint for themselves a governing body who are both entitled and obligated to protect the negative claim-rights of their citizens to life, liberty, health and private property.[9] By a 'negative claim-right' I mean the liberty of individuals to live, to be free, to remain healthy or to enjoy their private property without the illegitimate interference of others. Within the libertarian model, those in government should not take any redistributive measures – that is, they should not collect tax money from one group of people and then spend it to services which satisfy the needs of another group. This means that the state, such as it is, should not arrange any kind of socialized medicine, and that health care services ought to operate primarily on the principles of the free market, and secondarily on the basis of charity. Medical legislation is needed only to protect individuals against fraudulence and malpractice.

The core idea of *socialism*, at least in its democratic form, is that the working classes – or the majority – should form an extensive system of goverment which aims at securing everybody's positive claim-right to the equal satisfaction of vital needs. The purpose of socialist health care policy-making is to provide people with all the medical treatment – and other health-related services – that they genuinely need. When resources are scarce, as they frequently are in real life, the more basic needs of the population should be met first, leaving the more derivative and cosmetic needs, or desires, to be reckoned with in the future. In this model, all aspects of health care policy-making should be controlled democratically, that is, by the representatives of the people.

It is apparent that *some* people are regarded as moral experts in both libertarian and socialist ideologies. Libertarians state that moral choices should be left almost exclusively to those who pay for the services rendered by health care professionals and biomedical research groups. If I want to have contraceptives, or an abortion, or a cosmetic operation, or a lethal injection, my choice is limited only by my finances and by my capacity to find a physician who offers these services. If the board of a charity fund wishes to provide certain specified treatments to a certain specified group of people, the decision is theirs to make. And if the executives of a business enterprise endeavour to develop new gene-splicing techniques, they are free to proceed provided that they do not unduly threaten anybody's life, liberty or property in the process.

Socialist thinkers, again, tend to confine the right to make health-related moral choices to those who possess political or scientific authority. *Some* people have to define the needs that are, for the time being at least, more fundamental than others, and *they* must have a good idea of the structure and dynamics of social life, as well as sufficient knowledge concerning the physiology and psychology of the human race. Private citizens can often make ethical decisions when it comes to choices between treatment and non-treatment, or between two alternative lines of therapy. But these decisions take place in the framework of a centrally controlled health care system where nobody's needs are allowed, in theory, to trump anybody else's.

The problems of the libertarian and socialist models are, understandably, diametrically opposite, but as regards democracy they are on equally unstable footing. In the doctrine favouring individuals and their merits there is no room for people jointly caring for each other. This can easily lead to the glorification of selfishness, to the alienation of individuals from their fellow beings, and to the competition of everyone against everyone – not necessarily conditions under which a government of the people, by the people and for the people is likely to flourish. In the opposite corner, the ideology that prefers equality to deserts and moral or political constraints to freedom does not seem to provide individuals with an adequate opportunity to make autonomous decisions, as we normally understand them, concerning their own lives – not a very democratic-sounding solution, either.

The Communitarian Challenge

Many philosophers have during the 1980s and the 1990s chosen to believe that the main mistake of liberalism is its overstated respect for individuality, and that the most fatal flaw of socialism is its emphasis on the equal satisfaction of needs. These philosophers have found their spiritual home in *communitarian* thinking which combines meritism in the allocation of rights with collectivism with regard to the definition of freedom.

According to communitarian theorists like Michael Sandel,[10] Alisdair MacIntyre,[11] Charles Taylor[12] and Michael Walzer[13] liberalism is a skewed doctrine which should either be rejected or at least made to respect more traditional values than freedom and autonomy. They argue that human beings are not primarily individuals who are responsible for their self-determined choices, but members of their societies and communities, occupiers of their socially and culturally determined roles, and moral agents whose ethical values are defined by the linguistic and historical context in which they live. Liberalism, these theorists maintain, is an immoral view in that it does not recognize the need of human beings to belong to groups and to form their identities and ethical responses within these groups.

On the other hand, communitarian philosophers do not fully agree with socialist thinking, either. Sandel, for instance, in his critique of John Rawls, makes it clear that he rejects any form of the so-called 'communism of natural assets', that is, the idea that people can be justly made to use their talents and abilities for the benefit of others. (Rawls, by the way, far from being a socialist, is the great compromiser of our times, and his theories can be found right in the middle of Figure 7.1.) The critiques that MacIntyre and Taylor, in their turn, level at all types of reformism centre on the idea that while social and political institutions can change slowly and almost imperceptibly if they are allowed to develop without interventions, any human-made attempt to improve social conditions or political systems is condemnable and doomed to fail.

The communitarian idea of democracy seems to be that people's true opinions can be detected only by observing the traditional responses of their community to ethical issues. In health care policy-making this presumably means, in the affluent West at least, that the free market is permitted to reign in those medical matters which do not evoke strong adverse feelings among the population. As for the more controversial questions, policymakers probably ought to consult communitarian ethicists – theologians as well as philosophers – who are believed to be best acquainted with the morally genuine ideals prevailing in the society at large and in the smaller groups which together make up the whole.

It is completely incomprehensible to me that somebody can accept the communitarian model. There are two main reasons for my perplexity when it comes to health care policy-making. The first is that in many economically thriving societies communitarian theorists are prepared to leave their fellow human beings at the mercy of the free market in medical matters. The second is that in most tradition-oriented countries communitarians have to condone the nearly absolute subjection of the wishes of individuals to the paternalistic tyranny of the historical ethos prevailing in the society. This, again, can mean anything from the prohibition of contraceptives on religious grounds in Europe to the mutilation of the sexual organs of young girls for the sake of traditional values in the Middle East and in some parts of Africa.

The Liberal Egalitarian Alternative

My own intuition would be to go theoretically in the other direction, and combine needs-based positive claim-rights with the antipaternalistic, negative concept of liberty. The resulting view, which can be called *liberal utilitarianism*, states that individuals should be left free to make their own choices, provided that the consequences of their decisions are not likely to have a negative effect on the basic need-satisfaction of others. An important difference between the two types of egalitarianism depicted in Figure 7.1 is that while socialist thinking insists that people can and must be forced to be free, against their 'empirical wills' if this is ethically or politically necessary, liberal utilitarianism maintains that human beings can be to all intents and purposes free even if their actions are morally reprehensible. Another difference is that the liberal form of egalitarianism does not demand that people sacrifice their own basic need-satisfaction in order to satisfy the basic needs of others.[14] It can be true within socialism that the good of many should always preceed the good of one, but this is definitely not true in its liberal counterpart.

What distinguishes liberal utilitarianism from libertarianism is that in the former other people's needs are taken fully into account in ethical and political decision-making unless the fear of intolerable consequences to oneself prevents this. Well fed libertarians can walk through a crowd of starving people with their pockets full of bread without recognizing an obligation to share their food with others, but those who have taken to egalitarian ideals, even in their individualistic form, cannot.

In health care policy-making liberal utilitarianism, or liberal egalitarianism, stands for an extensive system of socialized medicine, accompanied with a zealous respect for the autonomy of patients and other users of the services. Democracy in this model means both concern for the well-being of the population *and* consideration towards the privacy and freedom of individuals. Health care systems which operate on these principles have been developed with varying degrees of dedication and success in the Nordic countries, and the most advanced example of policies which are at the same time liberal and egalitarian is without doubt Denmark.

Democracy and Morality

To answer the question of the title, then, does democratic might make right in health care policy-making within the four ideologies that I have sketched? Moreover, if it does, should it do so? In other words, is it morally justifiable to regulate choices in medicine and health care according to the will of the people as defined in the models?

I think that much confusion can be, and has been, caused by the fact that the answer to the first question is within all four views invariably and firmly affirmative. The decisions made by health authorities are, regardless of the background theory, morally improved when they, in some sense at least, take into account the 'voice of the people' in their work. The catch is, of course, that the sense in which the people's voice is important in one model can be quite alien to the ethos of the other doctrines.

Therefore, the more significant question concerns the moral legitimacy of paying attention to people's interests or opinions. With regard to this question, the views reveal their true natures and can be assessed more adequately. It is my conviction that the libertarian, socialist and communitarian theories fail to justify their appeals to the government or self-government of the people, because they do not, in the end, allow people – all people, the majority of people, or individuals taken separately – to become the true moral experts in health care decision- and policy-making. The libertarians are willing to listen only to people who are well-off, and can express their preferences and values by purchasing the services they want. Socialists profess to act in the best interest of people in general, but the way they define this goal can easily contradict people's own ideas of their own good. And communitarians make traditions and culturally determined habits and practices, rather than concrete, living and breathing individuals, the gatekeepers of the morally right and wrong.

The way liberal utilitarian, or liberal egalitarian, decision-makers take into account the opinions and interests of the people is twofold. At the first stage they try to define the most basic needs people have, and how these can be equitably satisfied in the society they live in. By basic needs I mean all those things which individuals must possess in order to be happy, or to have a good life. At the second stage liberal utilitarian decision-makers try to ensure that the autonomous choices of individuals are respected when they do not threaten the basic need-satisfaction of others.

The obvious practical problems of liberal utilitarianism include the definition of basic needs in an acceptable and informative way, and the solution of dilemmas created by conflicts of basic needs. There are many cases in which the moral guidance required must be sought by resorting to other principles. But the equally obvious advantage of this model is that it gives weight to everybody's interests and wishes in matters demanding moral expertise. Within this view people *are* the moral experts in medical related matters which concern themselves either individually or as a group looking for solutions which can be condoned as universally as possible.

I realize that, in spite of the title of this chapter, I have said nothing about democratic decision-making in the sense of voting, achieving majorities, securing the rights of minorities, forming coalitions, and the like. This is because I cannot see that kind of democracy solving any moral problems. Decisions often become more acceptable if they are made or supported by the majority, but they are not necessarily, I believe, rendered morally right by their popular appeal. This is why I have chosen to examine, instead, the role of the people in the four distinct normative archetypes of today's social and political philosophy.

Finally, my own solution, the liberal and egalitarian solution, is a combination of the views presented by Lady Caroline and Lord Illingworth. I agree with Lady Caroline in that public health authorities should provide people with blankets, coals and health rather than popular amusements. But when it comes to matters which concern only individuals themselves, I share Lord Illingworth's view that the uneducated people, if this is what they are after decades of exposure to health-related information, are the only ones who should have the right to vote.

Notes

The original version of this chapter was presented at the meeting *Who Are the Experts? - A Symposium on Ethical Expertise in Health Care*, Copenhagen, 15-16 June 1996. My thanks are due to Dr Søren Holm, who invited me to speak in the meeting and thus encouraged me to give a definite form to the ideas I had for some time had concerning the relevance of political ideologies in health care policy making.

1   *The Works of Oscar Wilde* (Leicester: Galley Press, 1987), p. 422.

2   *The Works of Oscar Wilde*, p. 422.

3   *The Works of Oscar Wilde*, p. 422.

4   *The Works of Oscar Wilde*, p. 422.

5   *The Works of Oscar Wilde*, p. 422.

6   *The Works of Oscar Wilde*, p. 422.

7   The distinction was made by Isaiah Berlin in his 'Two concepts of liberty' (originally published 1958), reprinted in: *Four Essays on Liberty* (Oxford: Oxford University Press, 1969).

8   This view is defended, e.g., in M. Häyry, *Liberal Utilitarianism and Applied Ethics* (London and New York: Routledge, 1994), ch. 3.

9   See, e.g., R. Nozick, *Anarchy, State, and Utopia* (New York: Basic Books, 1974); J. Narveson, *The Libertarian Idea* (Philadelphia: Temple University Press, 1988).

10   M. Sandel, *Liberalism and the Limits of Justice* (Cambridge: Cambridge University Press, 1982).

11   A. MacIntyre, *After Virtue* (London: Duckworth, 1981).

12   C. Taylor, *Sources of the Self* (Cambridge: Cambridge University Press, 1990).

13   M. Walzer, *Spheres of Justice* (New York: Basic Books, 1983).

14   Häyry 1994, ch. 3.

Printed and bound by CPI Group (UK) Ltd, Croydon, CR0 4YY

21/10/2024

01777086-0010